AF552727

Fat Rich Dairy Products

Foreword

Dairying has emerged as an instrument to bring about socio-economic transformation in the rural sector. The diversification of Indian Agriculture, as visualized by Planners, focused on dairying for sustainability and to meet future demands. A diversified segment of all section of farmers contributed to 120 MT of milk production, making India to become largest milk producer in the World.

During past several decades, India has developed infrastructure as well as expertise in tropical dairying. Efficient systems have been developed for procurement. Processing and marketing of wide range of western and ethenic milk products suited to tropical climatic conditions prevailing throughout the country and to economic development.

The emerging economic and technological forces are likely to further impact growth and development of dairying sector. Initiatives have been taken under the newly proposed National Dairy Plan to improve health aspects of milk and milk products, conservation of energy, Impact on environment, business and finance for sustainable growth.

The authors have interpolated their rich experience of academic and research gained at institutes of national and international repute in this book. Impressive endeavor have been made in documenting the basic principles of processing products rich in fat contents. The processing of fat rich milk products on the basis of applied aspects of chemistry, engineering and microbiology are essential in imparting sound understanding of the subject matter. The text book has been divided into nine chapters encompassing various techniques for processing, industrial practices and important grades, batch and continuous processes, packaging and most important the existing laws pertaining to quality assurance of such products. The book also deals in various techniques involved and practiced for testing the products for their quality parameters. This book will serve a useful reference for the undergraduate students pursuing dairy and food processing courses, teachers at various professional institutes and universities offering dairy courses, Planners and entrepreneurs.

Dr Oliver Brave
Ex. Head, Dairy Technology
Alld. Agri. Institute (SHIATS)
Allahabad, Uttar Pradesh, India

Fat Rich Dairy Products

D.K. Thompkinson
Sathish Kumar, M.H.

NEW INDIA PUBLISHING AGENCY
New Delhi – 110 034

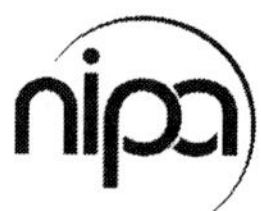

NEW INDIA PUBLISHING AGENCY
101, Vikas Surya Plaza, CU Block, LSC Market
Pitam Pura, New Delhi 110 034, India
Phone: + 91 (11)27 34 17 17 Fax: + 91(11) 27 34 16 16
Email: info@nipabooks.com
Web: www.nipabooks.com

Feedback at feedbacks@nipabooks.com

ISBN: 978-93-83305-80-3

Composed and Designed by NIPA

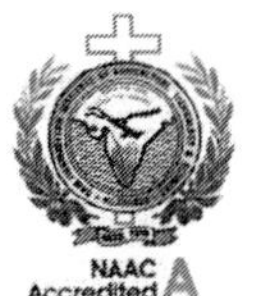

सैम हिग्गिनबॉटम इन्स्टीट्यूट ऑफ एग्रीकल्चर, टेक्नालॉजी एण्ड साइंसेज
Sam Higginbottom Institute of Agriculture, Technology & Sciences
(Formerly Allahabad Agricultural Institute)
(Deemed to be University)
Allahabad - 211 007, India
Established: 1910

NAAC Accredited A

ISO 9001:2008 Certified

मो० रेव्ह० प्रोफेसर राजेन्द्र बी० लाल, कुलपति
Most Rev. Prof. Rajendra B. Lal, Vice-Chancellor
Ph.D. Soil Science (Kansas State, U.S.A.)
P.D.F. Soil Environmental Quality (Kansas State, U.S.A.)
Ph. D. Ag. Botany (India)
FISAC, FBRS, GAMMA SIGMA DELTA Scholar

Office : 91-532-2684290, 2684284
Fax : 91-532-2684593, 2684394
Website : www.shiats.edu.in
E-mail : vicechancellor@shiats.edu.in

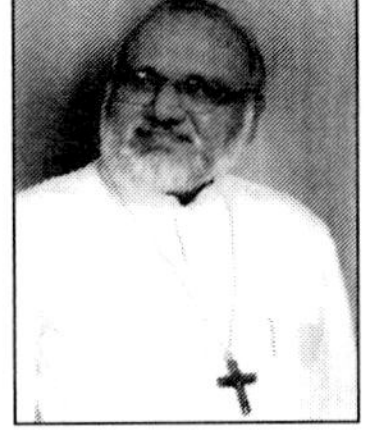

VC-467/Msg/20014/601

November 26, 2014

Message

The fear of the LORD is the beginning of wisdom, and knowledge of the Holy One is understanding.

Proverbs 9:10

India stands tall among the milk producing countries of World with an annual production of about 120 million metric tons. With recorded growth rate of 3-4% this is expected to touch 160 million tons by 2020. Milk being highly perishable commodity must be handled in a manner to preserve the quality of milk and derived products till it reaches the customers. During past several decades, India has developed impressive expertise and infrastructure in tropical dairying for processing and marketing of wide varieties of ethenic and western dairy products suited to economic conditions in the country. Newly emerging economic and technological forces are likely to impact further growth.

Indian dairy industry has been involved over several years, in converting surplus milk into various fat rich dairy products like butter, ghee and table spreads for technological, economical and environmental reasons. Nearly one third of total milk production is being utilized for manufacture of butter and ghee where milk lipids, an expensive constituent of milk, is concentrated and preserved. Dairy foods represent a major segment of the varied food industry. Milk lipids play a vital role in providing nutrition, flavor and textural attributes to dairy products.

Recent technological developments in dairy science has offered to have better control in existing processes and adopt noval approaches towards processing and quality assurance of existing and new products development. In advanced countries the dairy industry is diversifying its products that are specifically targeted in maintaining human health. There exist a vast opportunity to develop new milk products having improved nutritional and functional attributes.

This book has exhaustively covered various aspects of different fat rich dairy products encompassing their standards, manufacturing technologies, improved methodologies, packaging, storage, marketing, defects and usage and related quality assurance to safeguard human health. I found this book to be very useful for students, faculty members of various universities offering dairy courses as well as for existing dairy personals involved in routine processing and quality assurance operations.

I do hope that this book finds its due place and will prove to its usefulness in time ahead. My best wishes to the authors for their accomplishment and success in their endeavour.

27/11/2014

(The Most Rev. (Prof.) Rajendra B. Lal)

Vice Chancellor

Preface

This book has been written for the under-graduate students of Dairy technology course being offered by different Dairy Science Colleges and various Agricultural and Deemed Universities across the country. The need was felt to upgrade the only existing text, on the subject, to the collegiate for the last two decades. The book has been designed to cover the principles involved in processes and products that applies to dairy industry. Attempts have been made to categorically put forth the concepts of current technologies used for manufacture of fat rich dairy products and techniques involved in their quality assurance together, in an easily understandable expressions, for dissemination of information.

The topic covered under the text includes production and consumption pattern of fat rich products, about lipids specially milk lipids its composition and components and physico - chemical properties, various fat constants, processes and processing techniques for manufacturing of different fat rich produtcs, theoretical considerations, packaging, quality assurance and legal aspects including various food laws and implementation agencies involved during processing and marketing of milk products. It covers newer technologies available and being in use by different players in the dairy industry.

The book is a result of considerable experience by the authors in handling theoretical and practical aspects related to different courses in the subject of dairy technology as well as dairy plant operations. It is expected to be of value to the newly trained as well as existing technocrats engaged in Indian Dairy Industry.

Authors

Acknowledgement

The authors are indebted to the editors and publishers of variety of books and journals from which meaningful information has been gathered and compiled in this presentation. The authors are also gratefully acknowledge the contribution of their colleagues viz. Dr. Patel, Dr. Dharampal, Dr. Kanawjia, Dr. Aggarwal, Dr. Darshan Lal, Mr. Satish, Mr. K.L. Arora, Mr. Yogesh, Mr. Garg, Dr. Verma and Dr. Jessa Ram, at the department of dairy technology and dairy chemistry, who have from time to time shared their expertise in different aspects related to various techniques and processes, during preparation and presentation of this book into existing form.

The authors would like to express their deep sense of gratitude to Dr. B.N. Mathur, ex-Director, National Dairy Research Institute, Karnal for his valuable suggestions during compilation of subject matters and their presentation for this book. The authors are also indebted to Dr. A.K. Srivastava, Director, N.D.R.I., Karnal for his encouragement and permission to write this book.

The references from various books, journals, compilations, notes and presentations at the end of each chapter has been freely consulted, for which the authors are gratefully acknowledge the publishers and editors. Thanks are also due to our family members, well-wishers, friends and relatives for their continued support in this endeavor.

Last but not the least the authors extend their heartfelt thanks to the publishers of this book, since without their kind co-operation this book would not have seen the light of the day.

D.K. Thompkinson
Sathish Kumar, M.H.

Contents

1

Introduction

Several centuries ago, perhaps as early as 6000-8000 BC, ancient man learned to domesticate species of animals for obtaining milk for their consumption. These included cows, buffaloes, sheep, goats, and camels, all of which are still used in various parts of the world for the production of milk for human use. The significance of milk as the most wholesome single food available in nature has never been debated. It is as ancient as mankind itself. The role and consumption pattern of milk in the traditional diet varies widely in different regions of the world. The tropical countries have not been traditional milk consumers, whereas in Europe (especially Scandinavia) and North America, milk and milk products have been traditional parts of the diet.

Milk, an intricate combination of hundreds of different substances, and milk products have been explored and analyzed more than most foods. Technological advances have facilitated the alteration of milk processing from an art to a science. The availability and distribution of milk and milk products today in the modern world is a blend of the centuries old traditional knowledge of milk products with the application of modern science and technology. Certain novel characteristics of milk permit to extend its usage into innumerable forms. Milk may be concentrated, coagulated, fermented, fractionated into a vast range of milk products and derivatives, which is probably unmatched by nature's any other food. Milk may also be converted into products, which are more shelf-stable and to take care of the regional and seasonal fluctuations. India is the largest producer of milk (117 million tones) that consist nearly 55% of buffalo milk. Nearly half the milk produced is converted into various forms of milk products (inclusive of organized sector and private players). Buffalo milk is better suited for manufacture of fat rich dairy products because of its higher fat content, bigger fat globules, easier separation, lower loss in butter-milk and skim-milk and provides higher yield. Amongst the Indian fat rich products are – Malai, Makkhan, Cream, Butter and Ghee. Their counter parts abroad are – Cream (sterilized and frozen), Table butter and Butter-oil (anhydrous milk fat). India produces 28000–32000 tones of butter and 48000-54000 tones of ghee annually. Together they contribute about Rs. 23,750 crores to the Indian dairy sector. Many significant advances in the dairy industry have taken place during past decades contributing to the progress of dairy industry. The knowledge acquired has permitted better process control in handling milk and milk products. This may serve as a basis for development of new value added products for enhanced profits.

Table 1.1: Milk utilization pattern in India (percent)

Milk products	2004-05	2006-08	2008-10
Liquid milk	46.00	46.0	45.7
Milk powder*	3.0	3.6	3.5
Ghee	28.0	28.0	27.6
Butter	6.5	6.5	6.5
Khoa	5.5	5.5	6.5
Cream	0.5	0.5	0.5
Curd	7.0	7.0	6.9
Ice cream	0.7	0.7	0.6
Cheese**	2.0	2.0	2.1
Other	0.8	0.2	0.1

Compiled from different sources

Table 1.2: Butter production - major countries

Countries	Production ('000 tones)		Annual growth rate (%)
	2009	2010	
India	3855	4098	6.3
EU 27	1979	1968	- 1.3
USA	712	709	- 0.4
NewZealand	515	478	- 7.2
Russia	232	207	- 10.9
Pakistan	630	630	0.0

Source: FAO / IDF 2011. including butter-oil & ghee

Table 1.3: Butter production in India ('000 tonnes)

Year	Production
2005	2172
2008	3608
2009	3855
2010	4098

Source: FAO / IDF 2011 including butter-oil & ghee

Table 1.4: Fat rich product market (2007)

Catagory	Volume (MT)	Contribution (%)	Key players
Butter	35,500	9.0	Amul, Mother dairy, Britania, Nestle
Ghee	58,500	18.0	Amul, Nestle, Nova, Milk food, Haritage

Source: IDF, 2008

Milk Fat / Lipid

Commercially, fat is the most important constituent of milk. It is also the most variable fraction in milk. The percentage of fat in the milk of some of the breeds is as follows: Holstein, 3.5; Ayrshire, 4.1; Hariana, 4.8; Buffalo, 7.4. The percentage may vary with individuals of the same breed. The percentage variation is caused by many factors. Milk fat is present in the form of small globules (diameter: cow milk 3 to 8 micron, buffalo milk, 4 to 10 micron). The size and number of fat globules vary depending upon the breed of the animal and method of milking. The fat globules become smaller and more numerous as lactation advances. Machine milking produces fat globules of more uniform size than hand milking. Homogenization reduces the fat globules to a small size and reduces the tendency of separation during storage. The larger the size of the globules, the quicker they rise, as cream, to the top of the milk and easier it is to churn such cream into butter. For this reason buffalo milk lends itself to being churned into butter more easily than cow milk. The milk of animals in advance lactation is less suitable for being churned into butter. Milk containing small globules is, however, more suitable for cheese making since less fat is lost in whey. The composition of butter-fat varies with the feed plane of nutrition, stage of lactation, breed and species, the first being the most important. The melting points of different fats differ widely. That of butter, a mixture of different fats, ranges from 33° to 35.5°C. The normal body temperature of bovines being higher, the fat globules are present in liquid form in freshly drawn milk. Cooling milk to a little below the melting point of butter does not solidify the fat globules. The actual temperature below which the process of solidification would begin depends upon the relative proportion of individual triglycerides in butter as these have different melting points.

The colour of fat depends upon its carotene content and varies with the species, breed and feed of the animal. The yellow colour of cow milk is due to the carotene. Buffalo milk does not contain carotene. *Ghee* from cow fed on an abundant green fodder is more yellow than when fed on dry food. Similarly some breeds such as *Jersey* and *Guernsey* may produce milk deep yellow in colour. Milk-fat is quite bland in taste and imparts smoothness and palatability to fat-containing dairy products.

The mixed triglycerides make up to 98-99 percent of the milk fat. The combination of these triglycerides is peculiar to milk. Numerous triglycerides may be present in milk-fat, since milk contains as many as 437 different fatty acids. Typical are, butyric, caproic, caprylic and capric acids which are present in high proportions and are characterized by strong odours and flavour. These volatile fatty acids are not present in such high proportion in other naturally occurring fats. The fatty acid content of milk-fat can also be influenced by the amount and type of feeds consumed and also due to stage of lactation and the breed of the animal. Milk-fat also contains cholesterol, thus differentiating it from vegetable fats, which contain phytosterols. Milk contains 0.23 to 0.1 percent phospholipids, viz. lecithin, phosphatidy serine, sphingomyelin, inositol and cerebrosides. Some of these phospholipids serve as antioxidants in prolonging the shelf-life of fat rich product like *ghee.*

Milk Lipids - Physical Properties

At room temperature lipids are solid and are therefore, correctly referred to as "fat" as opposed to "oil" which is liquid at room temperature. Physical properties of milk fat have profound influence on textural and sensory attributes of fat rich dairy products like butter, ghee and table spreads. The viscosity of these products is also a function of physical state of fat globules. Crystallization and crystal state of globular fat play an important role in products like butter and table spreads. Crystallization of milk fat largely determines the physical stability of the fat globule and the consistency of high-fat dairy products, but crystal behaviour is also complicated by the wide range of different triglycerides. The process of crystallization consists of nucleation and growth phase. Crystallization starts with the formation of nuclei. The nucleation rate is increased by lowering of temperature. The growth of nuclei takes place by successive single layer of molecules that deposits on the already formed crystal surface. There are three well recognized form of crystals namely – α , β and β^1. Milk fat tends to exist in more than one crystal forms (polymorphism). This phenomenon causes milk fat to have multiple melting points. The melting point of milk fat is dependent on rate and temperature of crystallization. At a given temperature, milk fat that is cooled rapidly contains less liquid fat than the milk fat that is cooled slowly. Rapid cooling involves formation of relatively uniform crystals with similar melting point. The formation of mixed crystal influences the content of liquid fat in the mixture that greatly influences the rheological properties of resultant butter.

Refractive index is a valuable physical constant of milk fat and is the characteristic function of its fatty acid composition. Milk fat has a typical refractive index range of 1.453 – 1.457. The values of milk fat are lower than that of vegetable oils and therefore, forms a basis for detection of admixture of other fats and oils as judged by butyro-refractometer reading (BR reading) that ranges from 40 – 45 for pure milk fat.

The physical properties of milk fat can be summerized as follows:

Table 1.5: Physical properties of milk fat

Property	Value
Density at (20° C)	915 kg m(-3)*
Refractive index (589 nm)	1.462 (decreases with increasing temperature)
Solubility of water in fat (20° C)	0.14% (w/w) increases with increasing temperature
Thermal conductivity (20° C)	0.17 J m(-1) s(-1) K (-1)
Specific heat (40° C)	2.1kJ kg(-1) K(-1)
Electrical conductivity	<10(-12) ohm(-1) cm (-1)
Dielectric constant	3.1

Compiled from different sources

The four most abundant fatty acids in milk are myristic, palmitic, stearic and oleic acids. The first three are solid and the last is liquid at room temperature. The relative amounts of the different fatty acids can vary considerably. This variation affects the hardness of the fat. Fat with a high content of high-melting fatty acids, such as palmitic acid, will be hard. But on the other hand, fat with a high content of low-melting oleic acid makes soft butter. Determining the quantities of individual fatty acids is a matter of purely scientific interest. For practical purposes, it is sufficient to determine one or more constants or indices which provide certain information concerning the composition of the fat.

The melting points of individual triglycerides ranges from -75° C for tributyric glycerol to 72° C for tristearin. However, the final melting point of milk fat is at 37° C because higher melting triglycerides dissolve in the liquid fat. This temperature is significant because 37° C is the body temperature of the cow and the milk fat would need to be liquid at this temperature. The melting curves of milk fat are complicated by the diverse lipid composition such as trans unsaturation increases melting points where as odd-numbered and branched chains decrease melting points.

Table 1.6: Physico – chemical constant of milk fat

Attributes	Cow	Buffalo
Butyro-refractometer (BR) reading	41.2	42.0
Saponification value	227.3	230.1
Reichert-Meissle value	28.5	32.3
Polenske value	1.8	1.5
Krischer value	22.1	28.5
Iodine value	33.8	29.4
Melting point (°C)	28.5 – 41.0	32.0 – 42.5
Solidifying point (°C)	15.0 – 23.5	16.0 – 28.0
Colour (Yellow units/g) Tintometer	8.8	0.8

Compiled from different sources

Chemical Properties of Milk Lipids

The fat content of milk is of economic importance because milk is sold on the basis of fat. Milk fatty acids originate either from microbial activity in the rumen, and transported to the secretory cells via the blood and lymph, or from synthesis in the secretory cells. All fats belong to a group of chemical substances called esters, which are compounds of alcohols and acids. Milk fat is a mixture of different fatty-acid esters called triglycerides, which are composed of an alcohol called glycerol and various fatty acids. Milk fat consist of nearly 98-99% triglyceride (98.3%), small quantities of di and mono glyceride. Glycerol form the back bone of the triglyceride structure and the hydroxyl group of glycerol is esterified with fatty acids. The distribution of fatty acids on glycerol molecule could be inter or intra molecular. As triglycerides are synthesized in memory gland there exist some selectivity in esterification of different fatty acids at each position of glycerol moiety. There are approximately

437 different types of fatty acids identified from bovine milk. However, only handful of them are present in significant quantity and are of nutritional, chemical and physical importance. A fatty-acid molecule is composed of a hydrocarbon chain and a carboxyl group (formula RCOOH). In saturated fatty acids, the carbon atoms are linked together in a chain by single bonds, while in unsaturated fatty acids there are one or more double bonds in the hydrocarbon chain. Each glycerol molecule can bind three fatty-acid molecules, and all the three need not necessarily be of the same kind. The number of different triglycerides in milk is extremely large. The distribution of fatty acids on the triglyceride chain, while there are hundreds of different combinations, is not random. The fatty acid pattern is important when determining the physical properties of the lipids. In general, the SN1 position binds mostly longer carbon length fatty acids, and the SN3 position binds mostly shorter carbon length and unsaturated fatty acids. For example: C4-97% in SN3, C6-84% in SN3 and C18-58% in SN1 position.

The major fatty acids that contribute about 80% of total fatty acids are – butyric, stearic, myristic, palmetic and oleic. Milk fat is characterised by the presence of relatively large amounts of butyric and caproic acid. Table 1.7 lists the most important fatty acids in milk fat triglycerides.

Table 1.7: Principal fatty acids in milk fat

Fatty acid	Carbon no.	Cow milk (mole%)	Buffalo milk (mole%)
Butyric	C 4:0	3.3	4.1
Caproic	C 6:0	1.6	1.4
Caprylic	C 8:0	1.3	0.9
Capric	C 10:0	3.0	1.7
Lauric	C 12:0	3.1	2.8
Myristic	C 14:0	14.2	10.1
Palmatic	C 16:0	42.9	31.1
Stearic	C 18:0	5.7	10.2
Oleic	C 18:1	16.7	33.2
Linoleic	C 18:2	5.7	11.2
Linolenic	C 18:3	1.6	2.6
Arachidonic	C 20:0	1.8	-

Source: Gurr,1981; Arumughan,1978

Fatty acids are generally classified based on saturation (mono, disaturated or un-saturated); geometric isomerism (straight or branched chained) and chain length (small, medium, long). Amongst the saturated fatty acids butyric acid is prominent and unique of milk fat of ruminant animals as it is synthesized from diet in the rumen. Its importance is due to influence on flavour and off flavour of milk fat. It is responsible for the rancid flavour when it is cleaved from glycerol by lipase action. Saturated fatty acids are responsible for relatively high RM value and Polenski value of milk fat and soft texture and low melting point of milk fat.

Saturated fatty acids, such as myristic, palmitic, and stearic make up two thirds of milk fatty acids. Oleic acid is the most abundant unsaturated fatty acid in milk with one double bond. While the cis form of geometric isomer is the most commonly found in nature, approximately 5% of all unsaturated bonds are in the trans position as a result of rumen hydrogenation. Unsaturated fatty acids are of importance in milk fat as they contribute considerably to flavour, spoilage, chemical and physical properties. Depending upon the number of carbon atoms, poly-unsaturated fatty acids can either be termed as even or odd number fatty acids. They can further be classified based on their geometric isomer (cis or trans) or positional isomers (conjugated or non-congugated). Total content of un-saturated fatty acids in milk are about 34% and considerable proportion (10%) is in trans form. The small amounts of mono, diglycerides, and free fatty acids in fresh milk may be a product of early lipolysis or simply incomplete synthesis. Other classes of lipids include phospholipids (0.8%) which are mainly associated with the fat globule membrane, and cholesterol (0.3%) which is mostly located in the fat globule core.

Table- 1.8. Type of fatty acids in milk fat.

Saturated fatty acids	Mole %	Monounsaturated fatty acids	Mole %	Polyunsaturated fatty acids	Mole %
C 4:0	3.3	C 14:1	1.4	C 18:2	1.4
C 6:0	1.6	C 16:1	2.7	C 18:3	1.5
C 8:0	1.3	C 18:1	27.8	C 20:4	Trace.
C 10:0	3.0				
C 12:0	3.1				
C 14:0	14.2				
C 16:0	42.9				
C 18:0	5.7				

Source: Gurr,1981

Phospholipids : It is an minor constituent of milk fat that comprises to about 1% of the total fat. It is a important structural component of milk fat globule membrane surrounding the core triglycerides. They are esterified with fatty acids and phosphoric acid. Phospholipids are present in five major subclasses – phosphotidyl choline, phosphotidyl ethanolamine, phosphotidyl serine, phosphotidyl inositol and sphingomylene. The principal function of phospholipid is to maintain the milk fat in a finely emulsified state. They concentrate around the fat globules in the fat globule membrane and tend to stabilize the system. Phospholipid content of milk varies from 20 – 40 mg per 100g. The average content of phospholipids in cow and buffalo milk has been reported as 39.2 and 38.7 mg per 100g respectively. There is no appreciable difference in phospholipids content of different breeds of cows and buffalo. The phospholipids content of winter milk is higher than summer milk. Stage of lactation has significant effect on phospholipids content of milk. Colostrum is rich in phospholipids up to first week of parturition and thereafter is maintained at normal level. The level of phospholipids per unit weight of fat is 1.54 – 4.0 folds greater in fore milk than in residual milk. There is no marked difference in fatty acid composition of phospholipids from cow and buffalo milk fat. The major fatty acids of colostrums phospholipids are palmatic, stearic, oleic and linoleic. About 53% of total fatty acids are unsaturated. Cephalin is the most unsaturated fraction whereas Sphingomyeline contains mostly saturated fatty acids. Phospholipid content of cream increases with increasing fat content during mechanical separation of milk. During production of cream having 15-20% fat about 40% of original phospholipids goes to skim milk fraction. The final amount of phospholipids in ghee depends upon phospholipids content of butter and method of manufacture of ghee. Much of the phospholipids is lost in skim milk, butter milk and ghee residue. Phospholipids behave differently in aqueous and non aqueous systems. Milk phospholipids present in aqueous phase of milk triglycerides are relatively more stable and are preferentially oxidized. In dry products they act as anti-oxidants. Phospholipids possess chelating action on copper and display synergistic action with alpha-tocopherol.

Table 1.9: Phospholipid content of various milk products

Products	Cow (%)	Buffalo (%)
Milk	34.1 – 41.9	32.4 – 41.4
Cream	137.5 – 246.6	180.0 – 249.4
Butter	180.0 – 238.0	177.6 – 278.6
Butter milk	26.9 – 32.1	20.4 – 35.0

Compiled from different sources

Milk Fat Structure - Fat Globules

More than 95% of the total milk lipid exist in the form of tiny spherical droplets called fat globules, ranging in size from 0.1 to 15 μm in diameter, in the form of oil-in-water emulsion. Each fat globule consist of tri-glyceride (mostly) but a complex mixture of other lipids like- cholesterol, phospholipids, fatty acids, fat soluble vitamins are also associated with it. These components are present at the surface of fat globule. These liquid fat droplets are covered by a thin membrane, 8 to 10 nm in thickness, whose properties are completely different from both milk fat and plasma. The native fat globule membrane (FGM) is comprised of apical plasma membrane of the secretory cell which continually envelopes the lipid droplets as they pass into the lumen. The major components of the native FGM, therefore, are protein and phospholipids in the form of complex. There may be some rearrangement of the membrane after release into the lumen as amphiphilic substances from the plasma adsorb onto the fat globule and parts of the membrane dissolve into either the globule core or the serum. The FGM decreases the lipid-serum interface to very low values, 1 to 2.5 mN/m, preventing the globules from immediate flocculation and coalescence, as well as protecting them from enzymatic action. Milk lipids are found in three distinctly different phases of milk – fat globule, serum and fat globule membrane.

Table 1.10: Location of different lipids fractions in milk

Constituents	Range (%)	Location
Tri-glycerides	98 – 99	Fat globules
Phospholipids	0.10 – 0.20	Fat globule membrane
Sterols/cholestrols	0.25 – 0.40	All 3 phases
Free fatty acids	Traces	Serum / fat globules
Fat soluble vitamins	Traces	Fat globules
Vitamin A	7 – 8.5 mg/g fat	
Vitamin E	2 – 50 mg/g fat	
Vitamin D & K	Traces	

Compiled from different sources

Table 1.11: Fatty acids and tri-glyceride types of milk fat

Fatty acid and Tri-glyceride types	Cow milk fat (mole %)	Buffalo milk fat (mole %)
Total short chain (C:4 – C:10)	9.1	8.0
Total medium chain (C:12 – C:14:1)	17.1	13.9
Total long chain (C:16 – C:22)	72.2	76.4
High Molecular weight tri-glycerides	52.9%	42.4%
Medium Molecular weight tri-glycerides	18.9%	17.1%
Long Molecular weight tri-glycerides	28.2%	40.5%

Compiled from different sources

Buffalo milk fat: Buffalo milk is richer in fat content which contributes to its unique taste. The fat globule size is bigger than that in cow milk fat globule. Buffalo milk fat globule membrane contains 35% total lipids of which 72.44% are natural lipids and 16.86% are phospholipids. The natural lipid is composed of triglycerides of which 25.41% are low molecular weight and 27.27% are high molecular weight triglycerides. It also contains 4.56% monoglycerides, 6.92% diglycerides and 3.90% fatty acids. The average cholestrol content of buffalo milk is 20 mg / 100 ml which is significantly higher than that of cow milk. Buffalo milk fat differes significantly from cow milk in its fatty acid composition. It has higher proportions of butyric, stearic and palmatic acids and lower levels of caproic, caprylic, myristic and linoleic acids. Buffalo milk contain higher levels of tetraenoic and pentaenoic acids in its fat makeup. The total level of poly-unsaturated fatty acids (PUFA) and free fatty acids (FFA) are lower than in cow milk. The table below gives distribution of fatty acids on different triglyceride molecule between cow and buffalo milk.

Table 1.12: Percent Triglyceride distribution in milk fat

Triglyceride Type	Buffalo milk fat	Cow milk fat
SSS (trisaturated)	49.3	35.0
SSU (disaturated)	14.3	36.0
SUU (diunsaturated)	17.0	29.0
UUU (triunsaturated)	0.9	0.0

Source: Arumughan, 1978

Milk lipids rate high in their pleasing flavour that can not be duplicated by any other type of fat and which helps improve palatability. Milk lipid improves satiety value of diet, since fats stay in the stomach longer than do carbohydrates and proteins and is easily digestible. It is a carrier of fat soluble vitamins namely vitamin A,D,E and K and precursors of vitamin A and D. Milk lipids contain variety of triglycerides made up of saturated and unsaturated fatty acids, many of which are essential like Linoleic and Archideonic acids which are present in adequate amounts. Triglycerides are concentrated form of energy furnishing almost 9.3 Kcals. per gram of fat as compaired to 4.1 from carbohydrates and proteins. The short chain fatty acids are unique of milk lipids and are digested and absorbed quickly. The position of double bond linkages along the carbon chain in poly-unsaturated fatty acids , is important in nutrition. The position of unsaturation determines the point of break, along the carbon chain, during digestion process and thereby efficient absorption of resulting fragments through the intestine. Milk lipids also contain phospholipids and nitrogen along with fatty acids. Phospholipids are integral part of brain and nervous tissues. They are extremely important as intermediatory substance of fat metabolism. They play an important role in both human diet and nutrition. Lipids are necessary parts of all living tissues. They are vital components of brain and nerve cells and are essential to many physiological processes. They form reservoirs around vital organs and protect them against mechanical injury and are advantageous in stress situation.

Conjugated linoleic acids (CLAs) are a group of naturally occurring isomers of linoleic acid containing a conjugated double bond system. Different CLA isomers are present in milk and milk products from ruminant animals and are of great interest with respect to their anticarcinogenic effect. In fact, CLA is the only fatty acid that has clearly been shown to reduce cancer in experimental animals as well as in humans. A number of studies indicate that CLA inhibits human malignant melanoma and colorectal, breast, lung and ovarian cancer cell lines. Besides the anticarcinogenic effects of CLA isomers, they have also been reported to exhibit several biological activities such as reduction in atherosclerosis, increase in bone mass and muscle mass. They have also shown immuno-modulating properties. CLA isomers that originate from linoleic acids in the rumen are the major contributors to CLA in dairy products.

Suggested Readings

Arumughan, C. and Narayanan, K.M. (1978). Triglycerol composition of buffalo milk fat. J. Dairy Res., 19:81-85.

Arumughan,C. and Narayanan,.K.M (1978). Triglycerol composition of cow milk fat. J. Food Sci. Technol.,19:71-74.

Gurr, M.I. (1981). Review of the progress of dairy science. J. Dairy Res., 48: 519-554.

Jenness, R. and Patton, S. (1959). Principles of Dairy Chemistry. John Wiley & Sons Inc., New York.

Mathur, M.P., Datta Roy, D. and Dinkar, P. (1999). Text Book of Dairy Chemistry. ICAR Publ.

Morrison, W.K. (1970). Topics in lipid chemistry. Logas Press Ltd. UK

Palmer, L.S. and Samuelson, E. (1965). Fundamentals of Dairy Chemistry. AVI. Publ Co., USA. pp 442-444.

Pruthi, T.D., Naraynan, K.M. and Bhalerao, V.R. (1972). Fatty Acid Composition of Milk Phospholipids of Indian Zebu Cattle. Milchwissenschaft, 27: 294-296.

Walstra, P., Van Vliet, T. and Klock,W. (1995). Crystallization and rheological properties of milk fat. In: Advanced dairy chemistry-lipids vol. 2 second edition, (P.A. Fox, ed.) Chapman & Hall, London pp 179-211.

2

Cream

Definition

It is one of the important portion of milk which forms a fatty layer on top of milk when left un-disturbed. It is a prime component of milk and comprises mainly of milk fat. It may be defined as "that portion of milk which is rich in milk fat" meaning portion of milk into which larger portion of milk fat has been gathered. According to FSSAI, 2011 Malai and Cream are defined as –

Malai means the product rich in butter fat prepared by boiling and cooling cow or buffalo milk or a combination thereof. It shall contain not less than 25.0 per cent milk fat.

Cream including sterilized cream means the product of cow or buffalo milk or a combination thereof. It shall be free from starch and other ingredients foreign to milk. It may be of following three categories, namely:-

1. ***Low fat cream*** : containing milk fat not less than 25.0 percent by weight.
2. ***Medium fat cream*** : containing milk fat not less than 40.0 percent by weight.
3. ***High fat cream*** : containing milk fat not less than 60.0 percent by weight.

Note: Cream sold without any indication about milk fat content shall be treated as high fat cream.

Cream Powder means the product obtained by partial removal of water from cream obtained from milk of cow and/or buffalo. The fat and/or protein content of the cream may be adjusted by addition and/ or withdrawal of milk constituents in such a way as not to alter the whey protein to casein ratio of the milk being adjusted. It shall be of uniform colour and shall have pleasant taste and flavour free from off flavour and rancidity. It shall also be free from vegetable oil/ fat, mineral oil, added flavour and any substance foreign to milk. The product may contain food additives permitted in these regulations including Appendix A. It shall conform to the microbiological requirements prescribed in Appendix B. It shall conform to the following requirements:

(i) ***Moisture*** : Not more than 5.0 percent

(ii) ***Milk fat*** : Not less than 42.0 percent

(iii) ***Milk protein in milk solid not fat*** : Not less than 34.0 percent

Classification : Generally there are two basic classes of cream that are mostly recognized and these are:

A. ***Market cream*** : which is used for direct consumption like – table cream.

B. ***Manufacturing cream*** : which is used for manufacture of cream products.

Cream Production

Cream is generally produced by separating milk into its components – fat and solid-not-fat. These two basic components of milk can be separated out owing to the differences in their specific gravity. Milk fat being most expensive component, the recovery of fat is of importance in dairy processing because of its economic value. The pricing of milk is based on its fat content. Fat content of various dairy products need to be adjusted to meet the legal standards, before the milk is processed into product. The separation of milk into cream and skim milk is the foremost unit process to which the milk is subjected at the dairy plant. Milk separation is based on the principle of differences in the densities of fat (0.90-0.93), obtained as cream and solids-not-fat (1.027-1.032) obtained as skim milk. Milk fat therefore, has a tendency to rise to the surface. The technique used for separating one substance from another is a natural process of sedimentation by gravity. The substance to be treated must be a mixture of two distinct phases, one of which should be continuous phase. The phases to be separated must not be soluble in each other and they must also have different densities. Milk having serum part as continuous phase, which is heavier, and fat as dispersed phase, which is lighter, satisfy the requirements for separation of the two phases. The usual methods are gravity separation and centrifugal separation. Later method involves application of centrifugal force that acts horizontally and permits instantaneous separation of particles in accordance to Stokes Law, which explains sedimentation velocity.

Separation by Gravity (Batch Process)

Until the invention of centrifugal cream separator, cream was obtained from milk by the gravity settling process. The original technique used to separate fat from milk was by gravity, where the milk was left undisturbed in a vessel. The fat globules being lighter tend to move upwards and collect at the surface in the form of a layer of cream, which is skimmed off manually. The rate of movement of fat globules through the viscous fluid medium, under the influence of gravity, is determined by the diameter of the fat globule. In milk, fat globules exist in varying diameters ranging from 2–10 microns. Depending on the size of fat globule they take different time to rise to the surface in order to form the cream layer. This results in the process being slow and time consuming. The magnitude of sedimentation can be determined by physical quantities like particle density (Pp in kg/m3), particle diameter (d in M), density of continuous phase (P_l in kg/m3), viscosity of continuous phase (n kg/ m,s) and gravitation force (g = 9.81 m/s2). If the values of these quantities are known the sedimentation velocity of the particle can be calculated using the following formula.

$$Vg = \{d^2 (Pp - P_l) / 18\eta\}g.$$

where:

d = particle diameter

Pp = particle density

P_l = density of medium

η = viscosity of medium

g = gravitational attraction ($9.81 m.s^2$)

This indicates that the rate of sedimentation velocity of the particle can be influenced by three basic parameters namely - square of the particle diameter, differential densities between the phases and viscosity of continuous phase. The flotation velocity of a fat globule of larger diameter is higher than its counter part of smaller diameter. In reality fat globules cluster into larger aggregates and therefore, flotation takes place rapidly. Nevertheless, the process in itself is slow, cumbersome and time consuming. It also has lesser efficiency in completely separating all the fat from the milk. Three basic methods of gravity creaming of milk were in use earlier.

(a) ***Shallow pan method*** : A circular pan 18-24 inches in dia and 4-6 inch deep is filled two third with milk and left undisturbed in a cool place. Initially the cream rises fairly rapidly within a few hours but the smaller fat globules take a very long time resulting in incomplete creaming. The skim milk thus obtained contains 0.5-1.0% fat.

(b) ***Deep setting method*** : Here the milk is placed in metal containers 18-25 inches deep and 8-10 inch in diameter. The cans are filled with milk and placed in cold water. After 24 hours the skim milk is removed through a faucet provided at the bottom of the can. The skim milk obtained has 0.2-0.35% fat. The method has good control on cream quality due to lower temperatures involved and also may give fairly complete separation of fat.

(c) ***Water dilution method*** : The milk in this case is diluted with equal volume of water and allowed to set for 12 hours. The skim milk obtained has 0.3-0.4% fat. The method is based on the fact that by diluting the viscosity of milk is reduced and thereby the rate of rise of fat globules will be rapid. The method reduces the value of skim milk which becomes unsuitable even for animal feeding. It gives incomplete separation of the fat and does not have adequate control on temperature resulting in deterioration in the quality of cream.

However, none of the gravity separation system are suitable for large scale usage. A continuous gravity separation system is possible where the liquid is introduced from inlet side of the vessel, having certain capacity and flows towards the overflow at the other end. On the way the particles settle at different rates, due to their different diameters. It is possible to increase the area of sedimentation by inserting baffle plates in the vessel, which acts as separation channels. The sedimentation can proceed at the same rate but the total capacity of the vessel increases by the number of separation channels that determines the total available area for separation. A certain minimum channel width is required to avoid blockage of the channels that may occur due to accumulation of sedimented particles. With the invention of centrifugal separators gravity separation has been replaced with it.

Centrifugal Separation (Continuous Process)

When a vessel filled with liquid is spun around an axis a centrifugal force is generated that creates a centrifugal acceleration which is not constant like the gravity in the stationary vessel. The centrifugal acceleration increases with distance from the axis of rotation and with speed of rotation. The process can be used to increase the rate of sedimentation of particles having different diameters under the influence of centrifugal force. Here the centrifugal acceleration (rw2) is substituted for the gravitational acceleration (g) in the formula given above and can be used to calculate the sedimentation velocity of each particle in the centrifuge using the formula

$$Vc = \{d^2. (Pp - P_1)/(18\eta)\}\ rw^2$$

The use of centrifugal force to enhance rate of cream skimming mechanically paved the way for modern day centrifugal separators. The sedimentation velocity is 6500 times higher in centrifugal separation. It is possible to effectively regulate the fat content of cream using throttling valves placed over cream or skim milk out let of a centrifugal separator. This is to adjust the relative flow of liquids.

Let us see an example of flow of liquid through a cream separator. Cream represents nearly 10% of total through put.

Considering milk with 4% fat and through put of 20,000L/hr, the total fat passing through the separator will be

$$4 \times 20{,}000/100 = 800L/hr.$$

Assuming that 40% cream is required, the total amount of liquid discharge will be $800 \times 100/40 = 2000L/hr$

meaning 800L/hr of cream and 1200L/hr of skim milk

The cream separator is a mechanical equipment having a centrifuge bowl with baffles inserted in the form of conical discs. The discs with radial strips to keep them apart, rest on each other forming a separation channel. The disc stack is equipped with vertically aligned distribution holes. The milk enters through vertically aligned distribution holes at outer edge while the discs (80-200 nos.) rotate around the axis at high speed (10000-18000 rpm). The milk thus is subjected to centrifugal force acting on all particles. The portion having heavier density is forced towards the periphery and collected as skim milk to the space outside the disc stack. From there it travels through the channel between the top of the disc stack and conical hood of the separator bowl to a concentric skim milk out let. The cream consisting of fat globules, being lighter in density, rises towards the inner edge of the discs towards the axis of rotation and is collected separately. The high density solid impurities in milk settle outwards towards the periphery of the separator and collect in the sediment space. The sediment space volume depends on the size of the separator which is typically 10-20 liters. The solid that collects in the sediment space consist of leuocytes, hair, udder cells, straw and bacteria. The total amount of sediment may vary but could be about 1 kg for every 10,000 liters of milk.

For solid retaining type separators, it is necessary to dismantle the bowl manually and clean the sediment space at relatively frequent intervals. However, to save time and labour, the morden separators now are equipped with self cleaning or solid ejecting bowls for automatic ejection of accumulated sediment which is normally carried out at 30 – 60 minutes interval during the separation process.

Types of Cream Separators

The first centrifugal cream separator was made by a Swedish engineer Gustaf de Laval in the year 1890. This was equipped with especially designed conical discs. The number of discs however, changes in conjunction with the capacity of each separator. Initially small capacity of cream separators were made to handle 40–100 liters of milk at a time. These were hand driven machines having smaller bowl size. The bowl contains around 10–15 conical discs which make the disc stack. The bottom disc is caulked on both sides whereas the top disc has cream screw to control the fat content in resultant cream. Both cream and skim milk are collected through separate spouts fitted on top of the bowl. The milk supply is through a small tank fitted with a manually controlled tap. Such machines are generally tabletop type and used for handling small quantity of milk . Similar type of machines with motor driven facility are also available which are used for large handling of about 500 – 1000 liters of milk. These are much more efficient than hand driven machines and are self standing type. The bowl size is larger and may contain 20–50 discs of larger diameter than that of hand driven machines.

However, for commercial operations, where very large quantities of milk is to be handled the dairy, requires larger machines. These are generally motor driven and self standing type of machines equipped with disc stack having around

200-300 conical discs. These modern centrifugal separators are of two types - semi- open and hermatic.

Semi open design : Centrifugal separators with paring disc at the out let are called semi-open type. Paring discs are special outlet devices, where the rim of stationary paring disc dips into the rotating column of the liquid and continuously pares out certain amount. For preventing aeration of the product it is important that the paring discs are sufficiently covered with milk. In these separators the milk is supplied from the top through a stationary axial inlet tube. As the milk enters the ribbed distributor, it is accelerated to the rotational speed of the bowl before entering the separation channel in the disc stack. The centrifugal force throws the milk outwards to form a ring with the cylindrical inner surface. The heavier solid particles are deposited in the sediment space and the cream moves towards the axis of rotation to the cream paring chamber. The skim milk leaves the disc stack at the outer edge and passes between top disc and bowl hood to the skim milk paring chamber. The kinetic energy of the rotating milk is converted into pressure in the paring disc which is equal to the pressure drop in downstream line. The volume of cream discharged from paring disc separator is controlled by a throttling valve on the cream outlet. A given fat content in the cream corresponds to the given rate of discharge. An automatic constant pressure unit is fitted in the skim milk outlet to keep the back pressure constant. The cream outlet is adjusted to give the flow volume corresponding to the required fat content in cream.

Hermetic design : The milk in hermetic separators is supplied to the bowl through the bowl spindle. Here the milk is accelerated to the speed of rotation of the bowl and then continues to enter through milk distribution holes in the disc stack. The pressure generated by the external pump is sufficient to overcome the flow resistance through the separator. Hermetic separators are part of closed piping system. Automatic constant pressure unit is fitted with a diaphragm valve which is effected by air pressure during the separation process. If the pressure in skim milk side drops, the valve plug moves down wards and reduces the passage. This results in throttling which increases the skim milk pressure to the preset value. The bowl of hermetic separator should be completely filled with milk during operation to avoid any air.

The sediment discharge sequence may vary depending upon the type of centrifuge. Basically a fixed water volume is added to initiate drainage of balance water. The discharge sequence may be triggered automatically by a preset timer or manually by a push button. During separation process the sliding bowl bottom is pressed upwards against a seal ring by the hydraulic pressure from the water beneath it. When the water is drained from the space below the sliding bowl bottom it drops instantly and the sediment can escape. Fresh water is automatically supplied from the service system to close the bowl bottom tightly against the seal ring. The sediment discharge takes place in one tenth of a second. The sediment is discharged from the frame by gravity either directly into the sewerage or a vessel. For efficient cleaning of centrifuges large volume of sediment and liquid is discharged during each cleaning cycle.

Table 2.1: Characteristics of separation methods

Particulars	Gravity method	Centrifugal method
Nature of force used	Gravitational	Centrifugal
Speed of separation	Extremely slow	Very high
Operational scale	Small	Large
Fat percent in cream	10 – 25%	18 – 85%
Fat percent in skim milk	0.2% and above	0.1% or below
Total fat recovery	~ 80 – 85%	99 – 99.5%
Bacteriological quality of skim milk	Low	High

Controlling Fat Content of Cream

The centrifugal cream separators are equipped with a device for regulating the fat content of cream. It is actually a valve that reduces or increases the passage of cream or skim milk at their respective outlets. Depending on the location of the regulating device it may be termed as cream screw or skim milk screw. The volume and fat content of the cream can be controlled by tightening or loosening the cream screw. The moving of cream screw towards the center of the bowl causes a part of the serum, that would otherwise have gone with the cream, to be diverted to the skim milk out let resulting in higher fat content in resultant cream. Skim milk screw also produces changes in fat content of cream by changing the ratio of cream to skim milk. By moving skim milk screw nearer to the bowl center the amount of skim milk delivery is reduced and the amount of cream increased by added skim milk diverted to cream out let. In this way the fat content of cream can be varied within wide limits without affecting efficiency of fat recovery.

The percentage of fat loss can be calculated by following formula

$$\% \text{ fat loss} = \frac{\text{fat in cream - fat in milk}}{\text{fat in cream - fat in skim milk}} \text{ X } \frac{\text{fat in skim milk}}{\text{fat in milk}} \text{ X } 100$$

% fat recovery = kg fat in cream /kg fat in milk X 100

Yield of cream – The yield of cream may be calculated using the formula –

C = M x (fm – fs / fc – fs)

where

C = weight of cream in kgs

M = weight of milk in kgs

fm = % fat in milk

fc = % fat in cream

fs = % fat in skim milk

Factors Effecting Efficiency of Separation-(Fat Percent in Cream)

The centrifugal cream separator is an exceedingly efficient machine. It can recover almost 99% of the total fat in milk under normal operational conditions. This is in striking contrast to the gravity system of milk separation where only 80% of the fat is recovered. The efficiency of a separator in removing fat from milk, is generally measured by the fat content of resultant skim milk. Practically very low fat is present in skim milk portion of the milk if the milk is separated in a mechanically sound machine that is properly operated. Many cream separators in commercial usage produce skim milk containing not over 0.01% fat. Nevertheless, a number of factors are known to affect the efficiency of separation. Some of the common causes are:

Temperature of milk : In order to ensure greater efficiency in removing fat care should be taken to bring the milk at a temperature of 50 – 60 °C. There is little, if any, loss of fat in skim milk than separating it at lower temperature. The added advantage at high temperature lies in preventing excessive microbial growth. The modern machines are less subject to the effect of temperature but do show a somewhat higher fat loss in skim milk. The decreased efficiency at lower temperature results from slower movement of fat globules through the serum as a result of increased viscosity of cold milk. Also the cold cream has a tendency to stick to the bowl parts and move slowly towards the cream outlet resulting in clogging of the separator.

Acidity of milk : Normally, fresh bovine milk has acidity ranging from 0.14-0.16% lactic acid. The most common change in freshly drawn milk is formation of lactic acid due to bacterial action. The formation of acid, upto certain level, does not interfere with separation of milk as far as passage of fat globules through the serum is concerned. However, an appreciable amount of lactic acid, if formed, tends to bring about physico-chemical changes in the casein fraction of milk. Development of high acidity in milk results in coagulation of milk where casein particle move from soluble to insoluble state. At this point it is difficult to separate the milk. The particles of casein accumulate rapidly in separator slime causing frequent clogging and reduction in efficiency of separation.

Speed of separator bowl : Loss of fat in skim milk is certain if the speed of separator bowl is lower than that prescribed by the manufacturer unless the flow is reduced correspondingly. The speed of the bowl determines the amount of centrifugal force generated. In case of reduction in the centrifugal force due to lower acceleration, all the milk will not be subjected to centrifugal force and the net result is incomplete removal of fat from the milk. In separators where milk is drawn into the bowl by suction, it functions automatically to reduce inflow of milk with speed and thus avoid fat loss to a certain extend.

Rate of inflow of milk : The rate of milk inflow into the separator is important to control fat losses in skim milk. If milk travels through the separator too rapidly it is subjected to centrifugal force for a very short time and complete removal of fat becomes impossible. The rate of flow should be so adjusted that all the milk entering the bowl be subjected to centrifugal force. This would result in proper separation of the two phases in milk and complete removal of fat from the milk. For this reason separators are equipped with inflow regulating device so that correct flow of milk is ensured within fairly narrow limits.

Presence of air : If the milk indented for separation contains entrapped air bubbles it causes disturbance in the counter current streams of skim milk and cream between the discs and thereby lowers the efficiency of separation. The effect of air in the milk is greater with hermetic than open type separators. Semi enclosed separators should be operated with the float in feeder tank.

Fat globule size : The efficiency of separation is directly affected by the size of fat globules. The quantity of fat present as globules of 0-2μ in diameter go almost completely in skim milk. The greater proportion of fat globules of the size ranging from 2-3μ in diameter goes into the cream.

Clogging of bowl : During the separation process a gray sticky mass called as separator slime, accumulates on the wall of the bowl. This slime consists of mucilaginous material, dirt and bacteria that are thrown to the outer periphery of the bowl. As separation continues this wall may thicken enough to clog the separator bowl. This reduces the space between the bowl wall and the disc stack and result in remixing of flow of skim milk and cream thus reducing the efficiency of separation. The first indication of clogging is an increase in the flow of cream.

Mechanical condition of machine : The discs in the disc stack of the separator may occasionally become badly worn and out of shape due to continuous usage and mishandling. The badly worn discs result in incomplete removal of skim milk and cause remixing with cream thus affecting efficiency of separation. The other reason of reduced efficiency could be improper installation and leveling of the machine. In case the machine is not properly installed or leveled a vibration of the bowl occurs. This may result in remixing in the stream of cream and skim milk at some point during separation process and thus reducing the efficiency of separation. In setting up the separator the leveling of frame as specified by the manufacturer is important to avoid any vibrations in the machine.

Thermal Processing of Cream

Heat processing of dairy products is carried out with the objectives of enhancing the shelf life and make it safe for human consumption. Thermal processing is an integral part of food and dairy industry. Generally common pathogenic organisms are destroyed by mild heat treatment. However, heat resistant organisms require higher temperature and longer treatment time to be destroyed. Hence, thermal death point of such organisms have been made the basis for time-temperature combinations used for various thermal processes. The choice of this combination is a matter of optimization where both microbiological effect and quality aspects must be taken into account. The thermal destruction is concentration dependent and follows logarithmic order of inactivation. Thermal death rate may be defined as the number of cells destroyed in a given unit time. It is the time required to accomplish total destruction and is highly dependent on temperature and is specific for a given organism. The objective must be achieved with maximum retention of desirable characteristics such as colour, texture, flavour and nutrients.

Cream obtained from raw or pre heated milk is highly susceptible to spoilage and therefore has to undergo heat treatment to destroy the pathogenic microorganisms and inactivate the lipolytic enzymes so as to prolong its keeping quality and make it safe for human consumption.

Pasteurization : Higher fat content of cream tends to protect microorganisms from thermal destruction. Cream, therefore, is subjected to a more drastic heat treatment than milk to pasteurize it. With the holding method, it is heated to 63°C to 68°C for 30 to 60 minutes and with HTST method of 82°C to 87°C for 10 to 20 seconds. The cream should be cooled to below 10°C immediately after the heating process over a tubular surface cooler which also helps aerate the cream and remove some of its off odours, or cooled in a plate chiller.

Vacreation : In creameries it is more common to vacuum deaeration of cream, a process called "Vacreation", meaning heating the cream by direct steam injection to about 93°C under vacuum in a vacreator. This helps to deodorize it of volatile feed and weed flavours.

Sterilization : To increase the shelf life, cream is often sterilized in cans. The cream is standardized with skim milk to a fat content of 20 percent and preheated to 65°C. The cream is then homogenized at a pressure of 175kg per cm^2 in the first stage and 50kg per cm^2 in the second stage. At this stage, 0.25 percent citrate and 0.1 percent sodium tri-phosphate are added as stabilizers on the basis of weight of cream. The cream is then filled in 400g tins and sterilized at 120°C for 15 minutes in rotary sterilizers, followed by immediate cooling to below 38°C. The shelf life of sterilized cream is about 6 months. The product does not require any refrigerated storage but once the tin is opened it should be consumed within two days.

Alternatively, cream may also be sterilized by UHT processing followed by aseptic packaging. This process has facilitated availability of wide range of functional cream products that can be stored at room temperature for several months. UHT processing refers to heating cream to 135° – 150° C for 3-5 seconds. There are two major types of steam or hot water based continuous flow UHT processing system namely- Direct and in-direct heating system. In a direct heating system the standardized cream is first preheated to 75°-78° C before entering to final heater where steam is mixed directly into cream to achieve desired processing temperature. The mixture then flow through the holding tube. The pressure of saturated steam, at the entry point, is maintained corresponding to the sterilization temperature in the holding tube, through a pressure retaining valve. The heated cream then enters tangentially into a vacuum expansion chamber where excess of moisture is removed as well the cream is pre-cooled. The vacuum is so adjusted so as to evaporate same amount of water as added in mixing chamber. The product is then aseptically homogenized, cooled and packed in special multilayer packets called – Tetra-Pak. The in-direct heating system is similar to HTST milk processing. Both plate heat exchangers and tubular heaters may be used for heating purposes. Adequate plate profiles with wider gaps between plates are used to improve overall heat transfer rate and pressure drop. To avoid mixing of heated and non-heated cream in down stream regenerative section, higher pressure is maintained at downstream rather than upstream side.

Cream Products

The milk fat in cream may vary from 18-85% depending upon the purpose for which the cream is required. As discussed earlier cream may either be used for direct consumption or it may be used for manufacture of other fat rich products viz., whipped cream butter and ghee. Cream used for whipping and butter making usually contains 30-40% milk fat where as cream with 65-85% milk fat (plastic cream) is utilized for making ghee. In the cream, all the constituents of milk, viz., proteins, lactose, and minerals from original milk are proportionately reduced.

The approximate chemical composition of the categories of cream is given below:

Table 2.2: Composition of various type of cream products

Cream catagory	Fat content (%)
Table cream	20 - 25
Coffee cream / light cream	10 - 18
Sweet cream	25 - 30
Sour cream	28 - 30
Whipping cream	30 - 40
Cake cream	30 - 36
Plastic cream	65 - 85

Compiled from different sources

Table 2.3: Composition of different fat content cream

Constituents	Percent Fat contents		
	25	30	50
Water	68.2	64	54.5
Lactose	3.71	3.50	2.47
Ash	0.56	0.40	0.37
Solid-not fat	6.80	6.00	4.55
Total solid	31.8	36.0	54.5
Serum: Protein ratio	2.54	2.40	1.69

Compiled from different sources

Table cream

This contains 20 -25% milk fat and is used for direct consumption on table or may be used in whitening of coffee and tea. Such cream comes in pasteurized or sterilized form in Tetra-Pak cartoons and can be directly used. This cream is obtained by separating milk. The cream obtained is standardized to required fat content, homogenized at 200 and 50 bar in two stage homogenizer and then either pasteurized at 82° C for 15-20 minutes or sterilized using UHT process.

Sweet cream

This is obtained by separating fresh high quality milk and contains around 28% fat. It is prepared by standardizing the cream obtained followed by homogenization and pasteurization. The pasteurized cream is then filled into pre-sterilized containers and placed in cold room for cooling.

Coffee cream

It is a shelf stable product with a fat content of about 10-15%. The cream is first standardized to the required fat level, homogenized in a double stage homogenizer using pressure of 200 and 50 bar respectively and pasteurised at 90° C, filled into bottles, crown corked and sterilized in retorts. Alternatively, it may be UHT treated and filled aseptically into one way containers. Coffee cream must be homogenized which helps to prevent fat plug formation in the container. It also improves taste, whipping power and stability. Homogenisation has a direct influence on the flocculation stability of coffee cream in hot coffee, which is due to casein precipitation. Stability may be improved by addition of 0.02% sodium bi-carbonate. The stability can also be effected by acid in coffee, temperature of coffee and water used for making coffee (presence of calcium salts). There are two basic requirements which must be met in production of coffee cream. These are – the cream should be viscous and should be of high quality and good stability. It is necessary to select correct temperature and pressure of homogenization to obtain correct viscosity. The viscosity of cream increases with increasing pressure and decreases with increasing temperature. To achieve good result during homogenization, fat must be in liquid form. Coffee cream is generally packed in one way containers of standard net volume of 10 ml portions upto 200-250 ml capacity. Its key function is to whiten coffee but it may also be used in preparation of foods and drinks and for direct consumption. The important quality criteria are taste, whitening power and stability in hot coffee.

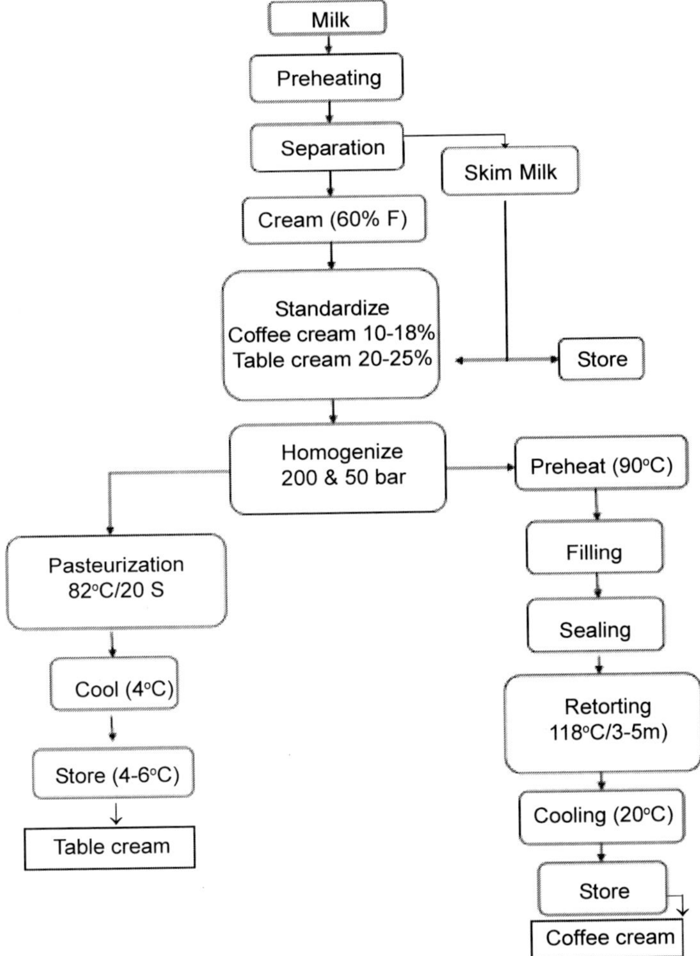

2.1: Schematic diagram for table and coffee cream

Sour cream

This is heavy bodied ripened cream of high acidity (0.6 percent lactic acid), clean flavour and smooth texture. It is made from sweet cream containing 18-20% fat. The cream is heated to 65° C and homogenized followed by pasteurization and cooling to 25° C. It is then inoculated with lactic acid culture @ 2-4% followed by incubation at 25° C and allowing fermentation to process until desired qualities are obtained (pH-4.5). It is then cooled to 2-4° C with gentle stirring, filled into suitable packaging containers and stored at low temperature until use. During fermentation, the homogenized clusters flocculate, resulting in highly viscous cream. To further increase firmness some times rennet or some other thickening agents are added to the sweet cream. Alternatively, in package fermentation process may also be applied. Sour cream is mostly used in prepared products such as salad dressing and tart toppings. The typical characteristics are white to yellowish and slightly creamy appearance, slightly acidic and clean flavour and sour taste. It is mainly used in prepared foods.

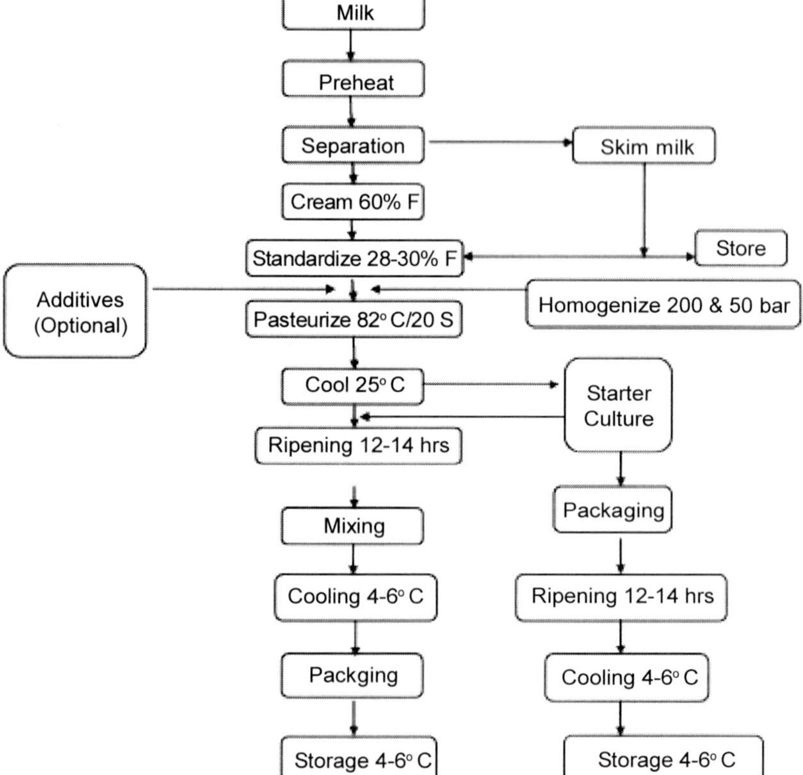

Fig. 2.2: Schematic diagram for manufacture of sour cream

Clotted cream

This cream product is exceedingly rich and contains around 60-70 % fat in a finally emulsified condition. It is prepared by heating cream to 78-88°C in shallow pans and then allowing it to cool slowly. The surface layer consists of clotted cream, which is skimmed off and strained. It has a peculiar boiled taste and rough appearance. Flavour and consistency depends on initial acidity of milk, time and temperature of scalding. The average composition of clotted cream may be 67.50% milk fat, 4.90% protein, 1.00% lactose, 0.50% ash and 26.10% moisture.

The Indian version of clotted cream is "*Malai lachha*". It is a heat dessicated clotted cream shredded into thin layers. It is pale yellow to light caramel in colour having delicious taste. High acidity milk may be used for preparation of Malai Lachha. Conventionally, both whole cow or buffalo milk or mixed milk may be used for the purpose. The milk is heated to concentrate using open pan vessel or steam kettle. The upper layer of cream is collected and allowed to cool. It is then cut into thin layers. Alternatively, cow or buffalo milk or mixed milk in the ratio of 1:1 to 3:1 may be concentrated using thin film scrape surface heat exchanger to attain up to 35-40% total milk solids. The concentrated milk is then allowed to pass through a lip slot die opening of 1.0-2.0 mm. As the clotted and concentrated product passes through the opening, a multi blade roller cutter cut the resultant product into uniform width. Finally the finished product is scraped with the help of scraper blade and collected. The *Malai Lachha* is used as a finishing material for garnishing of especially Bangali sweets.

Frozen cream

Cream is frozen to improve the keeping quality of cream during transportation over long distances and to store surplus cream for use during shortage. Mainly used by ice cream manufacturers who add sucrose (10-15 percent by weight) to cream before freezing to prevent oiling off after thawing. Frozen cream is obtained by separating and standardizing cream to 40-50 % fat; pasteurizing at 77° C for 15 minutes; cooling to below 4° C and filling/sealing into paper/plastic containers or tin cans. It is then frozen quickly and stores at -20° C or below.

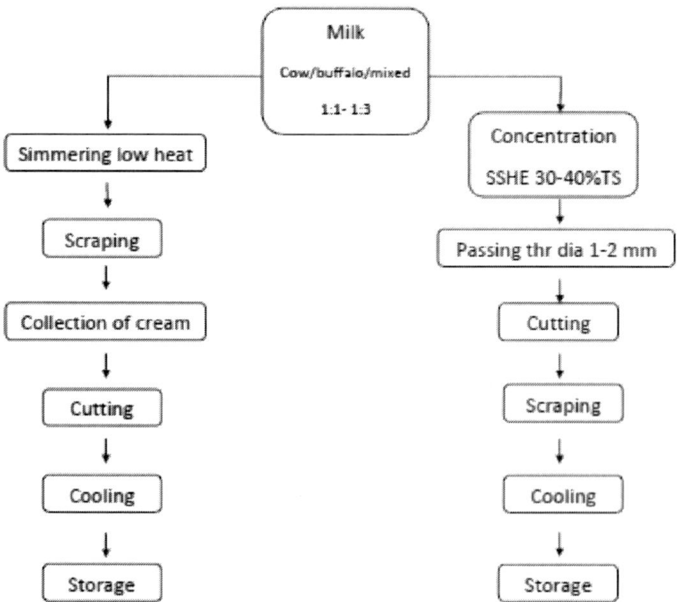

Fig. 2.3: Schematic diagram for preparation of clotted cream

Whipped cream

Whipped cream is a stable foam in which the air bubbles are entrapped in a mesh of serum and fat. To prepare a cream that will stand under its own weight and also look attractive, air bubbles is to be incorporated into it. Whipped cream is basically a food foam. It is prepared by standardizing the cream obtained to 30-40% fat to which sugar, emulsifiers and thickening agents (carrageenan) are added. The standardized cream is pasteurized at 80-95° C with holding time of 10 seconds before passing to the cooling section and finally to ripening tank. Here the cream allowed to further cool till 4-6° C and is held for at least 2-4 hours before agitation starts. Alternatively It may be processed and filled in pre-sterilized containers and stored at low temperature until final usage. Before final usage it is beaten or agitated into a foam to obtain desired body and texture.

During whipping air is intentionally incorporated into cream to produce froth containing small air bubbles. The fat globules collect on the wall of air bubbles. The mechanical treatment destroys the fat globule membrane librating certain amount of liquid fat which makes the globules to stick together. In order to get firm froth, fat globules must contain correct proportion of liquid and crystallize fat. Best whipping results are obtained when the cream is at or below 5° C and beating is constant and rapid. Whipping cream must be easy to whip and produce a fine cream froth with good increase in volume (overrun). The froth must be fine and stable and must not be susceptible to syneresis. This type of cream is mostly used as salad dressing and for decorating cakes. It is firm enough to retain shape during decoration and should not show leakage. It is also sold as ready made whipped cream in aerosol cans. It is available as a pasteurized product in small bottles, plastic cups or large cans. It is also sold as in package sterilized cream and even supplied with sugar and driving gas in an aerosol cans as ready made whipped cream. The desirable properties are:

Whippability : meaning that the cream should easily and quickly whip-up to form a firm and homogenous product containing 50% air (v/v) i.e. 100% overrun. To obtain firm foam the fat globules must contain correct proportions of liquid and crystallized fat. Best whipping results are obtained at temperature below 6° C. Normally 40% fat cream takes about two minutes to attain 100-130% over run and produce firm foam.

Stability : whipped cream should be firm enough to retain its shape and remain stable during decoration and should not show any leakage of liquid.

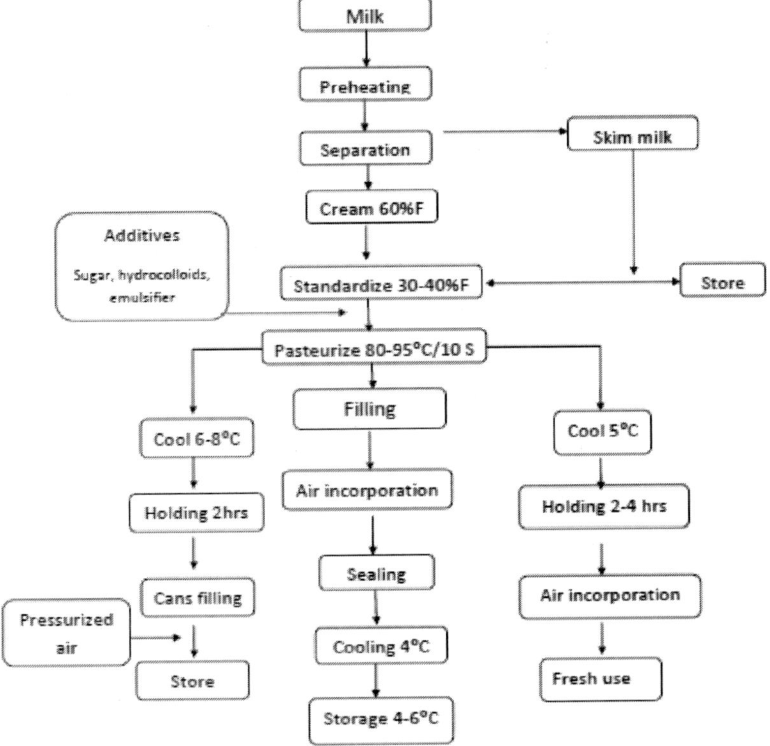

Fig. 2.4: Schematic diagram for manufacture of whipped cream

Whipped cream may also be obtained in powdered form as a free flowing powder with characteristic taste and creamy appearance. It is prepared by admixing powdered sugar, dried glucose syrup, hydrogenated vegetable oil, emulsifier, caseinates and modified starch. The maximum fat content is 70% and protein is 6.2%. The product is generally used for decoration of bakery products like cake by mixing 1.0kg powdered whipped cream in 1.5kg of water or milk at 5-8° C and mixed for 3-5 minutes.

Plastic cream

It is highly viscous than any other type of cream products. Its texture resembles to paste. This is obtained by re-separating normal cream (30-40 percent) in a normal cream separator, or separating milk in an especially designed plastic cream separator. In both the above cases, the initial product is pasteurized at about 71-77° for 15 minutes and cooled to 60-66°C before separation to get 75-85 % fat in the final product. It can be directly used for manufacture of ghee /butter-oil.

Sterilized cream

It is a product that is subjected to sterilization process in order to provide extended shelf life. The sterilization of product is attained either using in-package system or aseptic process. Fresh sweet cream is first standardized to 20 % fat and preheated to 80° C without holding. The cream is then homogenized at 250-300 bar and 50 bar in a double stage homogenizer. It is then immediately cooled to 16° C and filled in tin cans or glass bottles, sealed and sterilized using retort sterilizer employing at 118° C with 15 minutes coming up time, 10-12 minutes holding and 10 minutes for cooling at room temperature. Alternatively, the cream may be subjected to UHT treatment of 140° C for 3 seconds, followed by aseptic homogenization and packaging in Tetra-Pak of 200-250 ml capacity. Sterilized cream usually possesses a peculiar flavour and high viscosity with smooth texture.

Synthetic cream

It is basically a mixture of cereal flour, egg yolk, vegetable oil, sugar and water. Where egg yolk is not used it is replaced with any good emulsifier. The contents are mixed well until a homogenous mass is obtained. It is then heat treated, homogenized and packed in containers and stored until usage.

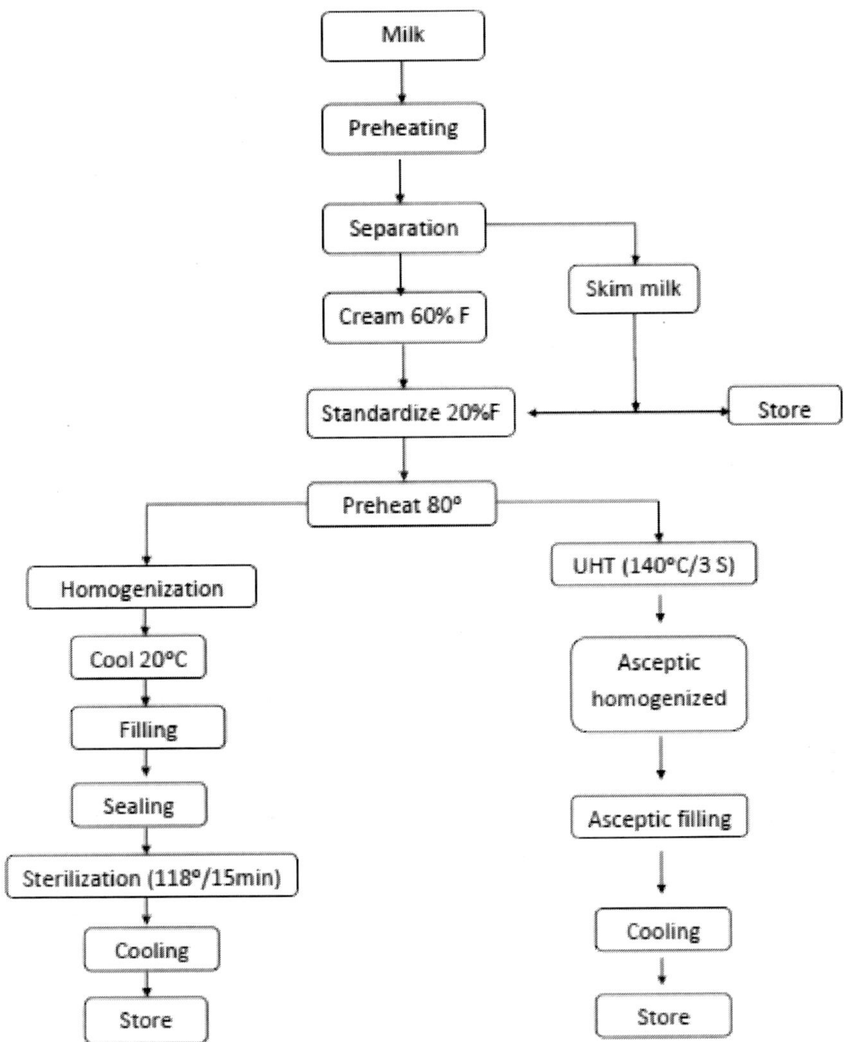

Fig. 2.5: Schematic diagram for sterilized cream

Cream powder

Cream may also be produced in powdered form by removal of water using suitable process. Such a product has greater shelf life. According to Codex standards (207-1999), Cream powder is a product which can be obtained by partial removal of water from cream. The fat and protein content may be adjusted, only to comply with the compositional requirements, by addition or withdrawal of milk constituents in such a way as not to alter whey to casein ratio of the milk being adjusted. Cream powder may be prepared using table cream as a starting material into which stabilizers (sodium or potassium citrate @ 500 mg/kg is added singly or in combination), Emulsifiers (Lecithin @ limited by GMP, mono/di glyceride @ 2500mg/kg and anticaking agent (Calcium phosphate, silicon oxide, magnesium/calcium/aluminium silicate @ 10,000mg/kg) single or in combination are added before drying. It may also contain antioxidants namely ascorbic acid or sodium ascorbate @ 500mg/kg expressed as ascorbic acid or butylated - hydroxy - anisol(BHA) @ 100mg/kg product. The chemical composition of such product is as follows:

Table 2.4: Composition of cream powder

Constituents	Level (%)
Milk fat (min)	42.0
Moisture (max)	5.0
Milk Protein (min) in MSNF	34.0

It is prepared by admixing all the ingredients in correct quantities and then the mixture is spray dried with an inlet temperature of 180° C and outlet temperature of 80° C. After cooling to room temperature, the fat rich powder in packed in 25 kg kraft paper bags with Polyethylene(PE) liners, for bulk packing and 200g to 1.0 kg packaging in lacquered tin cans which are sealed under inert gas (Nitrogen).

The BIS standards for fat rich dairy products are given below

Table 2.5: BIS requirements for cream & butter

Product	(Percent)				
	Fat (min)	Moisture (min)	Acidity (max)	curd (max)	NaCl (max)
Sterilized cream	20.00	-	0.15	-	-
White butter	82.00	16.00	0.06	1.50	Nil
Table butter	80.00	16.00	0.05	1.00	2.50

Cream Preservation

Cream being high moisture product is also highly perishable. In order to prevent spoilage of cream and to enhance its keeping quality, it is essential to process it as efficiently as possible after it is produced. The usual unit operations involved are thermal processing like pasteurization or alternatively it can be chilled and frozen. Pasteurization process (batch process), leads to increased air incorporation, high free fat content, plug formation and provides limited shelf life. Improved thermal processes includes-

1. ***UHT processing*** : For cream to be UHT processed it is first standardized to required fat percentage followed by pre-heating to 75°-80° C. It is then passed through the direct heating UHT plant where heating temperature is around 135°-150° C, using pretreated steam. After the holding period of 3-5 seconds it is passed through vacuum chamber where excess of water is removed and the cream is cooled before passing through an asceptic homogenizer. The cream is then aseptically packed and stored until usage.

2. ***In package sterilization*** : Here the standardized cream is first filled in sterilizable containers and sealed. The sealed containers are then subject to autoclaving/ sterilization to a temperature of 110°-120° C for 10-20 minutes followed by cooling and storage.

3. ***Freezing process*** : There are three different processes by which cream can be frozen

   a) ***Blast freezing*** : In this process cream is first standardized to around 40% fat, preheated, homogenized and finally heated to 80° C for 10 minutes, cooled and filled in pre-sterilized containers. After sealing the containers are shifted to blast chamber where they are instantly chilled. The containers are then stored at -20° C until further usage.

   b) ***Rotary drum freezer*** : Here the standardized liquid cream is kept in an shallow pan. A super chilled rotating drum picks up the layers of cream which freezes on the drum. Later at the end of rotation a knife is provided to scrape the frozen cream as cream flakes which is then packed and stored at low temperature (-20° to -30° C).

   c) ***Cryogenic tunnel*** : In this process the cream packages are placed over a conveyor belt and passed through a tunnel. Liquid nitrogen at -196° C is introduced into the tunnel where rapid freezing takes place by using latent heat of the low temperature boiling liquid (liquid nitrogen) to remove the product heat. The frozen cream thus obtained is stored at -30° C.

Suggested Readings

Bureau of Indian Standards, (1992). IS: 13690 -1992. Manak Bhavan, New Delhi.

Burton, H. (1988). UHT processing of milk and milk products. Elsevier Applied Science, London.

Dairy Technology – Principles of Milk and Milk properties and Processes. Editor – Walstra, P, Geurts,T.J., Nooman,A., Jellema, A. and M.A.J.S. van Boekel. (1999). Publ., Marcel Dekker Inc. USA.

De, S. (1980). Outlines of Dairy Technology. Pub., Oxford University Press, New Delhi.

Hinrichs, J. and Kessler, H.G. (1996). Processing of UHT Cream. IDF Bulletin N315.

Londahl, G. and Johanson, S. (1974). In-line freezing of cream XIX Intern. Dairy Congress, Vol. 1E, p. 649.

Milk and Dairy Products Technology, Editor- Edgar Spreer (1998). Publ., Marcel Dekker Inc. USA.

Modern Dairy Technology. Editor – R.K.Robinson (1994). Publ., Chapman and Hall, UK.

Towler, C. (1982) UHT sterilized coffee cream. XXI Intern. Dairy Congress, Vol.1, book 2, p.114.

3

Makkhan or Desi Butter

Introduction

Makkhan (Makhan) is an indigenous(*desi*) butter obtained by hand churning of dahi using wooden beater (*mathani*). It is traditional unsalted butter characterized by its delectable and rich flavour. It is white in colour with slightly greenish tinge and has typical soft body and a smooth grainy texture with pleasant aroma. This product has been extensively used for dietary and religious practices since vedic times. The entire quantity produced forms an intermediate product for preparation of ghee (clarified butter fat). Nearly 30% of the total milk production goes for desi butter manufacture. The average yield of the product is very low ranging from 5.5-7.0% for every 100 kg milk used for the purpose. The chemical composition of the product is variable depending upon the method of manufacture. It is difficult to achieve the uniform standard of 20% moisture in the final product due to limitations in the technique adopted for its manufacture. The non fatty solids and lactic acid are derived from the method of preparation and preservation. Higher non fatty solids in makhan indicates use of self soured milk, while a high lactic acid content indicates prolonged storage and in sanitary conditions of manufacture. Both these condition reflects poor quality and hence strict control of hygienic condition may assure better quality product. The average composition of the best product made under hygienic conditions shows 19-24% moisture, 76-84% fat, 1-3% non fatty solids and 0.20-0.50% lactic acid.

Method of Preparation

The art of converting milk fat into makhan is as old as the Vedas. The age old process is still continues even today in the rural India. The method of preparation is borne more out of experience than out of any scientific appreciation of the various factors involved. The reason for this status quo is the scattered nature of milk production and its unorganized utilization. In olden days when it was difficult for proper milk outlet, the farmer use to keep the left over milk in an earthen pot called "*chati*". Every day the left over milk is collected in *chati* until it is full. Generally it takes about 5-7 days for the *chati* to get full, depending upon its capacity that varies from 8-10 L. The collected milk under goes fermentation, during this period, and convert to dahi. This dahi is then churned with the help of mathani (wooden beater). The butter fat collected at the top of serum (butter milk) is collected by hand and stored in another container. The serum is also called " *lassi*" amongst rural populace and is used as a refreshing drink during summer season. The fat (desi makhan) collected fresh is used by the family members. The excess and that is collected from several lots of churning stored and later converted into ghee at convenient time.

The various steps involved during manufacture of desi butter, as is commonly carried out at villages around India, are enumerated hereunder with suggested improvements therof.

Raw material : Usually left over/unsold whole milk is used for the purpose. Buffalo milk is generally preferred but considerable amount of cow milk is also mixed depending upon type and number of animals raised by the farmer. The preference of buffalo milk is by virtue of its higher fat content that provides greater yield as compared to cow milk. The difference in yield may be attributed to differences in size and number of fat globules in both type of milk. Irrespective of the type of raw material used, it is desirable to have fresh and clean raw milk to have better quality of finish product.

Processing

Often raw milk is filled into the *chati*. Some times boiled milk is also added to the raw milk. Most commonly the raw milk is kept on low fire of cow dung as a fuel, and milk is allowed to simmer for 1-2 hours. It is then cooled at room temperature and filled into the *chati* and covered with a loose lid. Small lots of boiled and cooled milk are collected for several days before churning. As the village produced milk is generally contain higher bacterial load, due to unhygienic practices in milking, its finally affects the quality of resultant butter.

The undesirable influence of bacterial may be eliminated by adopting more suitable technique of heating raw milk to attain sufficient destruction of spoilage bacteria. This may help the desirable organisms to grow during fermentation process.

Curdling : This is a process to convert milk into curd before churning. The existing practice is to allow the milk to undergo natural souring. Generally the buttermilk from previous batch is used for the fermentation to take place. The period of setting generally varies from 12-48 hours. Where the milk is allowed to curdle naturally, the resultant butter is flat in flavour and of poor keeping quality. The loss of fat in buttermilk is higher and the yield of butter is low. Too low or too high acidity in curd is also not desirable for optimum yield and quality of final product. The inoculation of milk with good quality, active and clean lactic acid culture (*dahi*) free from mould and gas pockets may provide clean curd. The amount of inoculum may be adjusted according to the season of the year. Such adjustments can help to regulate the rate of acid development in milk. During hot summer season the rate of starter addition may be kept as 0.05-1.0% of the milk volume, whereas. during winter season when the temperature is low, it can be as high as 2.0-2.5%. As the time allowed for curd formation is governed by atmospheric temperature, The curd should not be over or under ripe at the time of churning. The optimum churning acidity of 0.7-1.0% is to be obtained within 8-10 hours in summer season and about 16 hours in winter season. The details of curding process includes, selection of proper starter for flavour and acidity development, time and temperature of curdling to ensure optimum acid production within normal time schedule (over night).

Churning : In rural setup the recovery of butter from curdled milk is usually carried out with the aid of wooden beater, called *mathani*. They come in various size and designs to which a long wooden pole is attached at one end. The beater is made to revolve in the container containing the curd clock and anti clock wise alternatively with the help of a rope wound around the pole. During churning there is no proper temperature control. Often water is added in varying amounts which serves to adjust the temperature and also lower the viscosity of curd for ease of churning. The process can take any thing from 30-50 minutes for the fat to separate out and accumulate at the surface of contents (serum). The violent agitation, produced by the *mathani* during churning, disintegrate the fat globules and increases the fat losses in buttermilk. Further, lack of temperature control prevents formation of butter grains and also adds to fat losses. The product produced is lumpy and is difficult to wash efficiently for removal of adhered buttermilk affecting the keeping quality of resultant butter.

An improved gear driven churn has been suggested for better recovery and quality product. The churn is fitted with a tap at the lower end to facilitate removal of buttermilk as well as wash water. The wooden beater is designed to have four pronged vertical baffle plates and connected to a gear drive for easy and effortless movement. The unidirectional motion of the beater helps in reduced time for churning and formation of granular butter. The temperature of churning can be controlled by addition of cold water directly into the churn. The water added should be equal to the quantity of curd churned. After the butter grain is formed, the buttermilk is drained through the faucet provided. The butter grains are washed with equal quantity of cold water for 5-10 minutes and the wash water is drained. The butter grains are tehn collected with a wooden scoop. Adopting these suggestions it is possible to enhance the recovery of milk fat to about 90% in the form of makhan. The product is likely to have better keeping quality.

Yield

The yield of makhan depends on the fat and moisture content as well as on the efficiency of fat recovery. It has been noticed that the out turn of makhan is numerically equal to the fat percent of original milk.

Table 3.1: Yield of makhan from different milk types

Type of milk	Average fat %	Yield	Kgs of milk needed for every 1.0 kg makhan
Buffalo	7.0	7.0	14.0
Cow	4.5	4.5	22.0
Mixed	5.8	5.8	17.0

Source: Srinivasan & Anantakrishnan,1964

Packaging

Generally the freshly prepared makhan, in small quantity, is collected and kept in a container for house hold usage. For commercial purpose small quantities of makhan is collected over a week and packed in tin containers of 15 kg size which is then sold to traders and transported to ghee clarifying stations.

Usage

Makhan is generally used fresh for serving at table for garnishing several vegetarian dishes like sarso-ka-sag, masala dosa, hot rice, steamed vegetables etc. It is also applied over chappati, stuffed parathas and makka-ki-roti. as a side dish

Future

Makhan or desi butter is usually made on cottage scale and lacks organized production and marketing. With the new trends in dairy development in the country it is believed that makhan industry may gradually disappear.

Suggested Readings

Acharya, K.T. (1998). A Historical Dictionary of Indian Food. Pub., Oxford University Press, New Delhi.

Anon (1990). Technology of Traditional Milk Products in Developing Countries. FAO Animal Production and Health Paper 85. FAO/WHO, Rome, Italy.

De, S. (1980). Outlines of Dairy Technology. Pub., Oxford University Press, New Delhi.

Srinivasan, M.R. and Anantakrishnan, C.P. (1964). Milk Products of India. Pub., Indian Council of Agricultural Research, New Delhi.

4

Creamery Butter

Butter is one of the leading milk product in developed countries of the world. It serves as a balance wheel of dairy industry. Surplus milk is generally converted into butter to be used during the times of scarcity. It is an article of commerce and a sign if wealth. Butter is a fat concentrate, which is obtained by churning cream, gathering the fat into a compact mass and then working it for proper distribution of moisture and salt. The art of butter making has a long history. The manufacture of butter was confined to colder regions where gravity creaming was successful. The milk was allowed to stand undisturbed for 10-12 hours until layer of cream collects at the top. The cream was then skimmed from top of the milk, taken into wooden tubs and butter made by hand churning. Later wooden churns were introduced where, following churning and discharge of butter milk, the grains of butter were collected in a shallow trough and manually worked until acceptable dryness and structure was achieved. The water content was dispersed in fine droplets through consistent working, so that the butter attains smooth consistency for easy spreadability and mouthfeel. Up to the middle of 19th century, manufacture of butter was mainly confined to the farm on cottage scales. Butter was originally made on the farm for household use which is similar to our desi butter or makkhan. Until 19th century butter was made from cream that is allowed to sour naturally. It was only after the development of centrifugal cream separator it became possible to skim cream before it became sour and thus butter could be made from sweet cream. Development of butter churn together with introduction of artificial refrigeration systems and pasteurization process around 1890, the industrial production of butter developed rapidly and large scale butter making in factories became possible during the later part of the 19th century.

Prior to 1970 most of the world butter was manufactured by batch process. Continuous butter manufacture was introduced around World war II to achieve increased manufacturing efficiencies. Regardless of manufacturing method employed, the essential feature of churning evolves destabilization of cream emulsion by means of mechanical agitation. About 6 percent of the total quantity of milk produced in India is used for making creamery butter in dairies and creameries. Today commercial butter making is a product of knowledge and experience gained over the years about issues like – pasteurization, hygiene, bacterial fermentation etc. as well as rapid technical developments resulting in advanced machines (continuous system) that are now available and used.

Definition

(i) ***General*** : Butter may be defined as a fat concentrate which is obtained by churning cream, gathering the fat into compact mass and then working it.

(ii) ***PFA, 2006*** : Butter is the product obtained from cow/buffalo milk or combination thereof, or cream or curd obtained from cow/buffalo milk or combination thereof, with or without addition of common salt and annatto or carotene as colouring matter. It should be free from other animal fats, wax and mineral oils, vegetable oils/fats. It must contain not less than 80% milk fat, not more than 1.5% curd and not more than 3% salt. Diacetyl may be added as flavouring agent not exceeding 4 ppm.

(iii) ***FSSAI, 2011*** : Butter means the fatty product derived exclusively from milk of Cow and/or Buffalo or its products principally in the form of an emulsion of the type water-in-oil. The product may be with or without added common salt and starter cultures of harmless lactic acid and / or flavour producing bacteria. Table butter shall be obtained from pasteurised milk and/ or other milk products which have undergone adequate heat treatment to ensure microbial safety. It shall be free from animal, body fat, vegetable oil and fat, mineral oil and added flavour. It shall have pleasant taste and flavour free from off flavour and rancidity. It may contain food additives permitted in these Regulations including Appendix A. It shall conform to the microbiological requirements prescribed in Appendix B. It shall conform to the following requirements : Moisture 16.0 percent m/m, Milk Fat- Table butter (80.0 per cent m/m), Desi/

cooking butter (Not less than 76.0 percent m/m) Milk solids not fat (Not more than 1.5 %), Common salt (Not more than 3.0 percent).

Provided that where butter is sold or offered for sale without any indication as to whether it is table or desi butter, the standards of table butter shall apply.

Legal Requirements

Butter is a fatty product derived exclusively from milk of cow and/or buffalo or its products principally in the form of an emulsion of the type W/O. The product may be with or without added common salt and starter cultures of harmless lactic acid and/or flavour producing bacteria. The butter shall be obtained from pasteurized milk and/or milk products which have under gone adequate heat treatment to ensure microbial safety. It shall have pleasant taste and flavour free from off-flavour and rancidity. It shall contain permitted food additives(Appendix-C). It shall confirm to prescribed microbial requirements (Appendix-D). Butter shall confirm to following requirements.

Table 4.1: FSSAI - requirements for Table and Desi butter

Constituents	Table butter	Desi butter
Milk fat (min.)	80.0 %	76.0%
Moisture (max.)	16.0%	-
Curd (max.)	1.5 %	-
Common salt (max)	3.0 %	-
Total plate count (max)	5000 / g	-
Coliform count (max)	5 / g	-
E. coli	Absent in 1.0 g	-
Salmonella	Absent in 25.0 g	-
Shigella	Absent in 25.0 g	-
Staphylococcus aureus	Absent in 1.0 g	-
Yeast and Mould count	20/g Max.	-

Table 4.2. Butter : Production, consumption and cost (2007)

Countries	Production ('000 tones)	Consumption (kg per capita/ annum)	Cost (per kilo)
European Union	1800	3.8	$ 3.2
America	400	2.2	$ 2.9
Africa	14	0.3	$ 2.7
Australia	150	3.2	$ 1.2
New-Zealand	360	2.1	$ 2.2
India (butter/ghee)	2500	1.8	Rs. 300
Canada	88.6	3.2	$ 4.6

Source : IDF, 2008

Type of Butter Products

1. Sweet cream butter (Farm butter)- 0.2% L.A.
2. Pasteurized cream butter (Creamary butter)-0.1- 0.15% L.A.
3. Sour cream butter – (made from ripened cream) -0.25-0.30% L.A.
4. Un-salted butter – no salt
5. Salted butter (Table butter) – with added colour and salt.

BIS Specification

Bureau of Indian standards has specified two types of butter namely-

A) ***Table butter*** : Means product made from pasteurized cream obtained from pasteurized cow/buffalo milk/combination with or without ripening with standard lactic culture, addition of common salt, annatto or carotene as colouring matter and diacetyl as flavouring agent.

B) ***White butter*** : Means the product made from pasteurized cream obtained from pasteurized cow/buffalo milk/combination without ripening and addition of any preservative, colouring matter and added flavouring agent.

Table 4.3: BIS – Standards (IS 13690:1992)

Constituents	White butter	Table butter
Milk fat (%)	82.0	80.0
Moisture (%) max.	16.0	16.0
Curd (%) max.	1.5	1.0
Salt (%) max.	nil	2.5
Acidity (% L.A.) max.	0.15	0.10
Coliform count (NMT)	5/ml	5/ml
Yeast & Mould count (NMT)	20/ml	20/ml
Diacetyl content (max.)	nil	4 ppm

Processing of Cream for Butter Making

1. ***Collection of cream*** : Butter may be prepared either from cream separated at the farm or cream separated from milk collected by the factory. Cream from farms are generally collected in cans from various routes where suppliers are numbered. The collection is done either by the factory itself or through contractors. The mode of receiving cream could be direct door delivery by the producers. In this mode of receiving cream problem may arise of regularity and quality of cream specially during summer season. Another way is to form cream stations at suitable distance and

cream produced in that area is collected at these cream stations which are maintained and operated by large creameries or is collected by local creameries. The cream collected in cans at these stations, on a particular route, are then transported through trucks to the factory. For long distance transportation of large quantities, cream in cans are transported by railway carrage or alternatively, it may be transported in refrigerated rail / road tankers.

2. ***Receiving cream*** : After reaching the factory, the cream is unloaded and samples are drawn for testing and grading. The process is similar as in case of milk. For all cream received in cans, the lid is first removed, inverted and sniffed to ascertain flavour. The cream is then checked for presence of any objectionable extraneous matter. The flavour of cream used for butter making plays an important role in influencing the quality of resultant butter. Many undesirable flavours may develop in cream. The general cause for off-flavours and odours may be (a) due to absorbed off flavour – which may appear because of longer exposure of milk/cream at the barn, resulting in Cowy or Barny flavour. The milk fat has the tendency to absorb volatile flavours rapidly and hence, milk/cream has to be kept in tightly covered containers away from foreign flavours/odours. Off-flavours like Mouldy, Yeasty, Putrid, Cheesy etc may also develop due to microbial actions causing souring in cream or putrification (protein break down) when stored at room temperature. Cream must be immediately cooled at 4° C before storage. Consumption of certain feeds giving off volatile substances/compounds may also cause off-flavours as such volatile compounds find their way into blood stream and finally into milk. Such flavours defects could be termed as Onion, Garlic, silage and Wild weeds flavours.

3. ***Grading*** : The grading is done on the basis of – acidity, time of delivery from production and quality. The outstanding considerations are – flavour and odour, presence of yeast or mould, age of cream (should not be more than 4 days under refrigeration), type of container, presence of foreign matter (insect, grass, sediment) and acidity. Cream is graded into 1st.grade consisting of sweet cream having acidity not more than 0.18% L.A. and 2nd grade consisting of sour cream having acidity more than 0.20-0.25% L.A. The quality of cream may be improved by adopting sound sanitary practices at the farm.

4. ***Weighing and sampling*** : All cans of cream that are accepted after grading are collected at one side and the cream is taken into standardization vat/ tank for further processing. Correct method is to weigh the individual lot before dumping into vat + amount of water from steaming of cans. Always measure cream when all of it is at the same temperature. Measuring cream quantity with calibrated metal stick may not provide accurate measurement, specially when cream contains considerable gas / air. Sampling of cream is done by mixing the can contents, thoroughly, with circular and vertical motions of plunger/agitator. In case the cream is thick/viscous, hot water is sprayed over the cans to reduce viscosity. A representative sample is drawn from different sections of can using cream dipper.

5. ***Testing*** : The composite sample of cream obtained are tested for Fat, Total solids and Acidity by standard methods. Both weighing and testing are important steps as correct methods will provide accurate amounts of fat and acidity present in a lot of cream. This will help in the process of standardization for fat as well as acidity required for butter making. The fat in cream is best determined using gravimetric method. The acidity is best determined in the fat free portion (serum) of the cream. For acidity test the cream is first heated to boiling temperature, cooled and then titrated against standard alkali.

6. ***Fat standardization*** : In the operation of a creamery, it frequently becomes desirable and some times necessary to standardize cream of any richness to a definate percentage of fat. This helps to minimize fat loss during

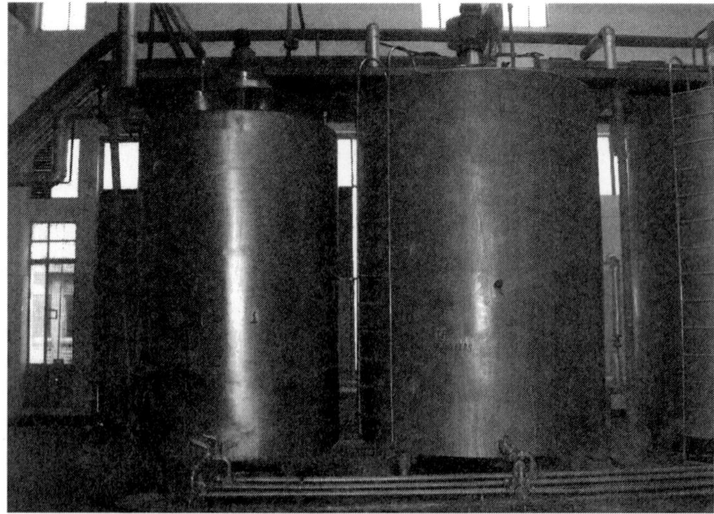

Fig. 4.1: Cream storage tank

butter manufacturing process. It refers to the adjustment of fat level in cream to desired percentage so that the final product confirms to requirements of legal standards. Fat in cream is usually adjusted to prescribed level by addition of calculated amount of skim milk. Generally Pearson's square method is applied for the purpose of standardization. The usual level of fat in cream is adjusted to 30-40% for butter making. Under Indian conditions cow milk cream may be adjusted to about 40% fat and buffalo milk cream is adjusted to about 35% fat. At this level of fat content, the viscosity of cream is low that could be churned easily leading to proper agitation and exhaustive churning that will help to reduce fat loss in butter-milk.

Pearson's square method : It is necessary to find the relative amounts of original and standardizing materials to be mixed together to give a product with desired fat content. Once the respective proportion have been determined it is easy to calculate the exact amount of each so as to mix together to provide certain weight of final product The proportions in which these raw materials are to be mixed to obtain required standardization is generally determined by Pearson's square method as follows:

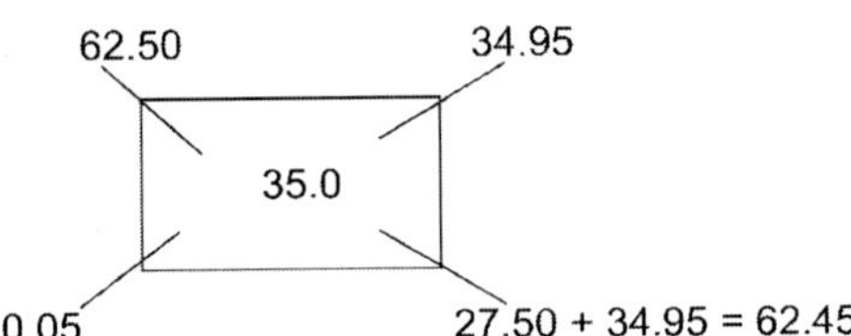

Here the fat percent of final standardized product is placed in the center of the square. The known fat content of raw material i.e. cream (62.50%) and skim milk (0.05%) are placed at the upper and lower left hand corners. Subtract the number in the center from the larger number at the left hand side of the square and place the remainder (27.50) at the diagonally opposite lower right hand corner. Similarly, subtract the smaller number from the number in the center and place the remainder (34.95) at diagonally opposite upper right hand corner. The numbers on the right hand side represent the number of parts of each of the original material that must be blended to make a product with the fat test given in the middle of the square. In above example the figures 34.95 and 27.50 at the right hand corners corresponds to the parts of cream and skim milk respectively to be used to secure 35.0% fat standardized cream. If the numbers on the right side are added, the sum obtained (62.45) will represent the parts of finished product with the fat test given in the middle of the square.

The example indicates that if 34.95 kg of cream containing 62.50% fat is mixed with 27.50 kg of skim milk containing 0.05% fat will provide 62.45 kg of standardized cream which will contain 35.0% fat.

Proof

62.45 kg of 35.0% cream contains 62.45 x 35.0/100 = 2185.75 kg fat

34.95 kg of 62.50% cream contains 34.95 x 62.50/100 = 2184.37kg fat

27.50 kg of 0.05% skim milk contains 27.50 x 0.05/100 = 1.37 kg fat

Now add kg of fat supplied from cream and skim milk

2184.37+ 1.37 = 2185.74 kg

(which is equal to the fat content of 62.45 kg standardized cream). This validates the calculation.

7. ***Neutralization*** : This refers to partial reduction of cream acidity. It is an important part of butter making where acidity should be reduced sufficiently so that the resultant butter has satisfactory flavour and texture. If butter is to be stored for several months, neutralization to an acidity that will give butter serum pH value of 7.0 is most satisfactory to preserve original flavour of butter and avoid storage defects. For short storage period the ideal churning acidity should range from 0.13% - 0.15% L.A. for medium and low acid cream and 0.17% - 0.18% L.A. for high acid cream.

The reasons/objectives of standardization of cream acidity are:

a) To control fat loss during churning- pasteurization of sour cream causes coagulation of casein thereby entrapping fat globules. As bulk of the curd goes into butter-milk, it causes high fat loss.

b) To control flavour of butter- Butter made from sour cream and salted develops fishy flavour.

c) To control keeping quality of butter - Salted butter made from sour cream can not be stored for long period with out development of off-flavours.

d) To manufacture butter of uniform quality each day having desirable texture.

It is advisable to follow correct method of neutralization as improper method and over neutralization both are deleterious to the flavour and keeping quality of butter.

Procedure

1. ***Adopt definite standard for churning acidity*** : Every factory has its own standards for adjusting cream acidity required for butter making depending upon weather the butter is to be consumed fresh or stored for long periods. The best range of cream acidity for butter making is 0.14-0.16% L.A. as it causes no problems with respect to off-flavour development, short or long time storage and gives butter of appropriate quality. However, for butter that has to be stored for longer period, the cream acidity should be reduced to 0.06-0.08% L.A. before churning. Where butter is intended for early consumption (not to be stored long) the acidity of the cream may be adjusted to around 0.20-0.25% L.A.

2. ***Correct testing*** : The acidity of cream is mainly because of the serum portion and therefore it is advisable to determine cream serum acidity. This refers to the acid content in fat free portion of cream. Serum acidity is more reliable than cream acidity. The acidity reduction should therefore be based on acid present in serum. Exact acidity in cream may be calculated by multiplying the acidity with 100 and dividing with the serum value (Example - 0.25 x 100/70). The serum portion may be calculated by substracting fat percentage from 100 (100 – fat). Secondly, it is always best to heat the cream to boiling to remove CO_2 dissolved in cream. This CO_2 acts as carbonic acid and increases the titratable value during testing and may result in over neutralization.

3. ***Amount of neutralizer*** : To calculate the amount of neutralizer to be added to a vat of cream one must know:-

   a) ***Correct amount of cream in the vat*** : To calculate the amount of neutralizer to be added, it is important to know correct amount of cream available for neutralization. Generally cream is measured using a calibrated metal stick but it may not be accurate in case of gassy cream. It is best to weigh each lot before dumping into the vat.

   b) ***Amount of lactic acid to be neutralized*** : For correct neutralization it is necessary to make correct weighing and testing of cream in order to know the exact amount of lactic acid that needs to be neutralized. This step helps towards selection of correct neutralizer and its amount required for proper neutralization.

c) ***Type of neutralizer to be used*** : Generally there are two groups of neutralizers that are available for the purpose. These are "LIME" compounds like calcium hydroxide (Ca(OH)2), magnesium hydroxide (MgOH), mixture of calcium hydroxide and magnesium oxide and mixture of calcium oxide and magnesium oxide (quick lime). The purity, solubility and reaction speed is low of Lime neutralizers. However, they are economical in use because of their low cost. Lime neutralizers combine slowly with lactic acid. Some of it combines physically with casein, increases cream viscosity specially in high acid cream and produces mealy texture in butter. It is required in higher quantity for neutralization. Second is the "SODA" compounds like sodium hydroxide, sodium carbonate, sodium bicarbonate and their mixture called sesquicarbonate. Some times modified or special alkali consisting of mixture of sodium hydroxide and sodium bi-carbonate in the ratio of 60:40 is also used for lowering acidity to 0.4% followed by use of milder neutralizer. Soda neutralizers have high solubility, purity and reaction speed. Soda neutralizers combines rapidly with lactic acid and provide better control for acidity adjustment. It does not cause thickening of cream and thereby less dangerous to cause scorched flavour and injury to butter texture. However, exclusive use of sodium hydroxide may give soapy flavour to butter as it forms soap with fat.

d) ***Amount of neutralizer required*** : To know the amount of neutralizer needed to partially reduce acidity to the required standard one needs to calculate the amount of lactic acid present in given amount of cream. To calculate how much neutralizer type is required to neutralize 1.0kg lactic acid, divide the molecular weight of neutralizer type by the molecular weight of lactic acid. Assuming that the molecular weight of lactic acid is 90 and that of sodium bi-carbonate is 84, the requirement of sodium carbonate will be 84/90 = 0.93. This means 0.93 parts of sod.-bicarbonate will neutralize 1.0 parts of lactic acid. Accordingly, depending upon the amount of lactic acid present the amount of neutralizer type can be calculated. Theoretically about 0.41kg of lime neutralizer and 0.93 kg of soda neutralizer is required to neutralize 1.0 kg lactic acid. But in practice these values are 0.49 and 0.85-0.91 respectively.

This difference is due to actual neutralizing capacity of lime being only 80%. The lower value for soda neutralizer is owing to the presence of varying carbon di-oxide. Meaning proportional decreasing effect of CO_2 with rise in cream acidity.

Table 4.4: Solubility of different neutralizer types per 100 ml water

Neutralizer type	Cold water	Hot water
Calcium hydroxide	0.185 g	0.077 g
Calcium oxide	0.131 g	0.070 g
Sodium carbonate	7.1 g	45.5 g
Sodium bi-carbonate	6.9 g	16.4 g
Sesqui-carbonate	13.0 g	42.0 g

Table 4.5: Amount of neutralizer type required to neutralize 1.0 kg lactic acid

Neutralizer type	Amount (Kg)
Sodium carbonate	0.63
Sodium bi-carbonate	0.93
Sodium hydroxide	0.44
Sesqui-carbonate	0.77-0.85
Sodium hydroxide + sod.carbonate (60:40)	0.50
Calcium hydroxide	0.50
Cal.hydroxide + Magnesium oxide	0.38
Cal. Oxide + Mag.oxide	0.30

Table 4.6: Neutralizer factor (NF) of different neutralizers
(part of lactic acid neutralized per part of neutralizer)

Neutralizer type	Neutralizer factor
Sodium carbonate	1.70
Sodium bi-carbonate	1.10
Calcium hydroxide	2.43
Magnesium hydroxide	3.10
Sodium hydroxide	2.25

Calculation

1. First of all decide upon the desired churning acidity (say-0.15% L.A.).
2. Determine serum acidity of the cream (say- 0.45% L.A.)
3. Decide upon the type of neutralizer to be used.
4. Calculate reduction in acidity required (0.45-0.15) = 0.30%

5. Multiply this with the amount of cream to know the amount (kg) of lactic acid present that needs to be neutralize.
6. Calculate the amount of neutralizer required by dividing its molecular weigh with the molecular weight of lactic acid as is described above.
7. Alternatively, multiply the reduction in acidity required with the neutralizing value required for 0.01% acid in 100 kg cream.
8. Now multiply this value with the total amount of cream in a batch.

Quantity of neutralizer = (a-b) (wt. of cream)/100 x NF

a = initial acidity and b = desired acidity, NF = neutralizer factor

Lime neutralizers should be weighed accurately and mixed with 10-15 times its weight of warm water. For making stock solution make sure that each liter of solution will neutralize definite amount of lactic acid. The stock solution is diluted with water before addition to cream. Soda neutralizers are weighed accurately and dissolved in 15-20 times its weight of water.

Double neutralization : This means where cream acidity is reduced by using two different types of neutralizers. This is done for cream having excessive acidity exceeding 0.65% L.A. Both lime and soda neutralizers are used to avoid neutralizer flavour effect that may arise due to use of large amount of single neutralizer and to avoid excessive carbon-di-oxide production by use of soda neutralizer for high acid cream. It is advisable to first use lime neutralizer for reducing about one third (1/3 rd.) acidity in a high acid cream, to a level of 0.30-0.40% L.A. The remaining two third (2/3 rd.) acidity is reduced by using soda neutralizer to the desired level of 0.15-0.20% L.A.

Correct addition of neutralizer : Accurately weigh the calculated amount of neutralizer type and dissolve in 15-20 times its volume of warm portable water. Heat the cream slowly to around 32°-36°C. Keep the cream agitated while adding the neutralizer solution uniformly and quickly. Continue agitation for next 5-10 minutes. Check the acidity by drawing representative sample. Finally pasteurize the cream at 78°-80°C for five minutes, immediately cool to 4°C and store overnight.

The problems encountered by using neutralizers are : thickening of cream, mealy texture in butter and pronounced limey flavour in butter where lime neutralizers are used. Where as soda neutralizers create excessive production of CO_2 during heating of cream and may result in over flowing in batch process of heat treatment. However, this can be reduced by dissolving the neutralizer in hot water. They may also produce definite soda/soapy flavour in butter when used exclusively.

Over neutralization : This means addition of excessive neutralizer to the cream than required. This may be the result of improper assessment of quantity of cream in vat, using more than the required amount of cream for acidity test, not removing carbon-di-oxide from sour cream before testing, using weak alkaline solution for acidity test, use of incorrect strength (too strong) of neutralizer, improper calculation and weighing of neutralizer salts.

Causes of Neutralizer Flavour in Cream

- Wrong assessment of amount of cream
- Improper acidity determination
- Incorrect calculation for neutralizer addition
- Adding more than calculated amount of neutralizer
- Reducing acidity below standard
- Adding neutralizer to cold, lumpy and heavy cream
- Use of too concentrated solution of neutralizer
- Using single neutralizer for high acid cream
- Improper addition of neutralizer

Pasteurization

In food manufacture public health aspect demands foremost consideration. Thermal processing is an integral part of food and dairy industry. The main purpose of heat treatment is to render the product safe for human consumption and to enhance its shelf life. The basis behind heat treatment is the destruction of micro-organisms and enzymes that cause spoilage. The common pathogenic organisms are destroyed by mild heat treatment. However, heat resistant organisms require higher temperatures and longer time to be destroyed. Hence, the thermal death point of such organisms have been made the basis for time-temperature combination used for thermal processing that could be achieved by various means. Pasteurization, as applied to butter making, may be defined as a process of heating cream to a temperature sufficiently high and for a duration of time sufficiently long to ensure destruction of micro-organisms present in the cream followed by prompt and efficient cooling to 4°C or to the ripening temperature. Efforts to ensure maximum germ destruction consistent with minimum heat flavour have let to the establishment of following recognized methods:

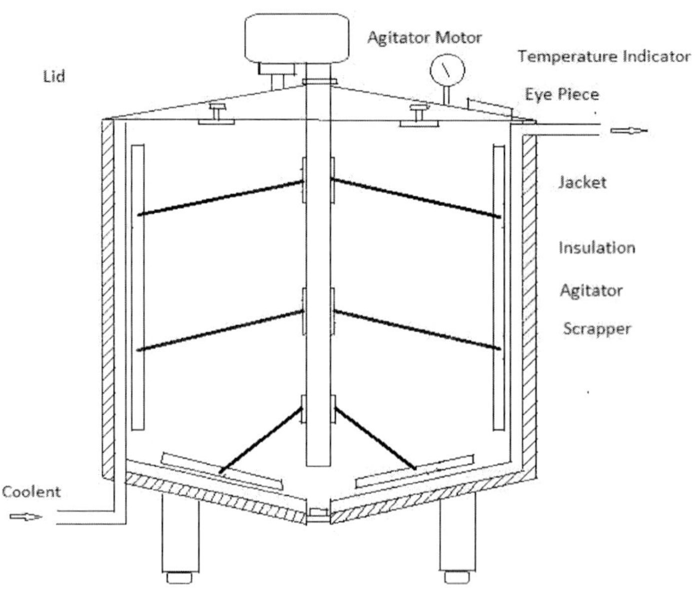

Fig. 4.2: Cream processing tank

1. ***Holding method*** : This is a batch process where 100-300 kgs of cream can be processed at a time. The process is also known as low temperature long time (LTLT) technique. Here the cream is held in a vertical tank equipped with coils to carry heating or cooling medium and a agitator on top of the tank to keep the cream agitated during the process. The cream is heated by batch system to 68°-74°C and held for a period of 30 minutes, followed by batch cooling. Alternatively, a circulation system may be attached to a vat through which the cream is recirculated via heating/ cooling plates.

2. ***Continuous methods:*** the process is also called high temperature short time (HTST) which is carried out in plate heat exchanger (PHE). The cream is allowed to pass through series of plates between which the heating medium is passed in a counter current. The cream is heated to a temperature of 78°-82°C for 20-25 seconds followed by immediate cooling, in the similar faction, before storing at 6-8°C.

3. ***Flash pasteurization*** : This is an continuous system where the cream flows in a continuous stream through the pasteurizer and is heated to 85°C or higher followed by flash cooling.
4. ***Combination of both*** : Here the cream is heated by continuous method to 72°-78°C and held in a vat for 20-30 minutes, followed by batch cooling.

The standards established for pasteurization of cream for butter making are capable of destroying micro-organisms with thermal death point higher than those of disease germs.

Effect on keeping quality : The keeping quality of butter is controlled by two distinct forces namely, bacterial activity and chemical reactions. They may be inter-related or dependent upon one another or may be independent or antagonistic to each other. Efficient pasteurization that accomplishes a low bacterial count improves general keeping quality of butter and also prevents development of specific bacterial defects like- rancidity or surface taints, caused by specific organisms. Pasteurization is a controlling factor in keeping quality of un-salted butter stored at temperatures above freezing point. Even presence of 2.5% salt in butter does not make the butter immune to damaging bacterial contamination. It may still develop rancid and putrid flavour defects. Efficient pasteurization is the only way to protect against these defects.

Effect on flavour : Efficient pasteurization intelligently adjusted tends to benefit butter flavour. It is improved partially due to expulsion of objectionable volatile flavours and partially due to destruction of organisms. This makes possible the effective control on fermentation between pasteurization and churning. Sour neutralized cream can be converted into butter without serious flavour damage, provided that the heat exposure, heating up and cooling down is done quickly and the cream churned within 1-2 hours after cooling.

Effect on body and texture : Excessive long exposure to heat and too slow cooling of cream causes butter with a "mealy" texture. The body and texture of butter can be improved by using efficient pasteurization temperatures and methods.

Effect on fat loss : Pasteurization of sour cream increases fat loss in butter-milk. This is due to entrapment of fat in curdled particles. As the bulk of the curd passes into butter-milk the fat so entrapped is also lost. In general high temperature tends in the direction of higher fat loss than lower temperatures of heating.

Ripening of Cream

Butter may or may not be made from cream that has been ripened. Ripening refers to the fermentation process which has been defined as the metabolic process where chemical changes occur in organic substrate like – protein, carbohydrate or fat through action of enzymes librated by specific living organisms. Lactic acid fermentation is the most important fermentation in dairy industry. The ripening of cream requires starter culture of suitable strain (single or mixed) capable to bring about fermentation (biochemical conversion of product components) which are closely dependent on the properties of starter culture involved and the type of product made. The major objective is to produce butter with a pleasant, pronounced characteristic flavour and aroma through out the year. The formation of diacetyl is essential for products like butter, fresh cheese, cultured cream, cultured butter-milk etc.

Starter is basically a culture of one or more types or strains of lactic acid bacteria that is added to milk or cream to ferment it. Traditionally it is obtained via growth of lactic acid producing bacteria in skim milk at a suitable temperature. It is subsequently maintained by propogating and growing in fresh portions of milk or special growth medium. There are two major types of starter organisms that are used for cream ripening, namely – a) Single strain starter culture consisting of a strain of *Lactococcus lactis ssp. Cremoris / Lactococcus lactis ssp lactis biovarient diacelactis.* And b) Multi strain culture containing strains of *Lactococcus lactis* ssp *cremoris* and or *lactis*. Often combination with biovarient *diacelactis* or with *Leuconostoc cremoris* and *Lactococcus lactis*.

Starters used for diacetyl formation are generally aromatic type. In such starters the ratio between the bacterial strains involved are very critical. The initial number of *Lactococcus lactis* ssp *cremoris* should not be too low as it may result in low number of aromatic bacteria in the final product. Whereas, the *luconostoc spp* should not be too high. These bacteria form diacetyl at low pH.

Streptococcus Family

1. ***Homofermentative*** :

   a) Streptococcus

   b) Lactococcus - *Lactococcus lactis* ssp *lactis, Lactococcus lactis* ssp *lactis* ssp *cremoris.*

   c) Pediococcus

2. ***Hetrofermentative*** : *luconostoc* spp

Their growth temperatures are minimum 8°-10°C and maximum 22°-28°C and they form diacetyl and or acetyldehyide. The rate of addition should be 0.5-2.0% and the incubation is carried out at 21°C for a period of 14-16 hours. The flavour intensity in butter depends on its diacetyl content. Butter with 0.2-0.6% diacetyl content is characterized as mild flavour. Full flavour can be obtained when diacetyl content is in the range of 1.5-2.5%. However, it should not exceed 4.0% as per legal standard.

Cooling and Aging of Cream

The process serves as an intensive preparation of cream for churning. Ageing is basically a time- temperature process to which the cream is subjected. It serves to restructure the liquid fat into crystalline state which is the basic requirement for solid, plastified structure of butter. Cooling and aging influences the criteria like consistency, firmness and spreadability of butter ; water content of butter and fat content of butter-milk. Butter is W/O emulsion and the fat globules in butter contain a considerable part of crystalline fat. The firmness of butter may be effected due to – composition of fat which has considerable effect and can be affected by type of feed and season of the year. Secondly, it may also be affected by the temperature treatment given to the cream during the cooling period. Slow cooling due to low heat transfer co-efficient favours formation of solid structure due to changes in crystallization which proceeds slowly if less liquid fat is available. The most important characteristic of butter is its sufficient firmness but it should be easily deformable in mouth without being greasy and melt quickly.

Fat is a triglyceride and its melting/crystallization behavior depends on type of fatty acids which provides an indication of hardness of butter. Natural hardness is caused mainly due to seasonal feeding. Feeding of dry feed yields hard fat with higher percentage of saturated and short chain fatty acids. While, feeding of green fodder results in larger proportion of unsaturated fat with longer chain fatty acids. Optimal fat crystallization has a decisive influence on butter formation. The type and means of crystallization kinetics can be influenced by temperature profile of cream. Once the fat is in range of melting/solidifying temperature, any further reduction in temperature disturbs the solution equilibrium of fat molecules and may result in super saturated state of the solution. As a result initially small crystals are formed which grow with large crystal structure. During crystallization a fractionation of fat takes place in stages. The higher melting fractions attach themselves below the membrane in the form of crystalline shell. The solidified fraction is mixed with liquid fat and semi-solidified fat in from of gel spheres. There are four different fat globule type fractions that may occur during cooling of cream at 11°-15°C.

1. Fat globules with a thin peripheral crystal layer and a liquid interior.
2. Fat globules with a thin peripheral crystal layer as well as crystalline fat agglomerates + liquid fat. – (This combination will result in harder butter).
3. Fat globules with a thick crystalline shell and a liquid core.
4. Fat globules with a thick crystalline shell and crystalline agglomerates + liquid fat. (This combination will result in softer butter)

To have butter of desired consistency it is important to control fat crystallization during cooling process. Consistency is a concept involving properties such as hardness, viscosity, plasticity and spreadability. It is one of the important characteristics as it effects taste, flavour and aroma of resultant butter.

The fatty acid composition of milk fat varies with type of feed and season. The relative amount of low and high melting points of fat makeup is a deciding factor towards hardness/softness of the butter. The ratio of liquid to solid fat is high when the milk fat contains high concentration of low melting fatty acids, that result in high content of soft fat. Whereas, when the ratio of liquid to solid fat is low, the resultant fat is hard. The consistency of butter is therefore, decided by the chemical composition of milk fat. Soft milk fat will result in softer and greasy butter. Whereas, hard milk fat will produce hard and stiff butter having poor spreadability. After pasteurization the fat in fat globules is in liquid form. When cream is cooled to 40°C the fat starts to crystallize. During gradual cooling, different fats will crystallize at different temperature as per their melting points. Gradual cooling results in minimum solid fat crystal formation but takes longer time that may make the milk fat sensitive to bacterial attack.

Quick cooling of cream to low temperature can speed up crystallization process. However, low melting point fat is trapped in the same crystal leading to formation of mixed crystals. The ratio of liquid to solid fat would be low and the resultant butter would be harder. To avoid this, the cream must be carefully heated to melt low melting triglycerides out of the crystals. The melted fat is then re-crystallized at a slightly lower temperature in order to obtain softer fat having higher ratio of liquid to solid fat.

If the milk fat is of hard type, the amount of mixed crystals must be minimized and pure fat maximized to increase the ratio of liquid to solid fat in the cream. To achieve the result following steps are performed :

1. Rapid cooling at 8°C and holding for two hours.
2. Gentle heating to 20°-21°C, using hot water at 27°-28°C and holding for two hours.
3. Cooling to about 16°C.
4. Final cooling to churning temperature of 8°-10°C.

Cooling Process

To obtain desired characteristics in butter and to maintain its consistency day to day it is important to control the cooling/ageing process. This has special significance when feed is changed depending upon the seasons. This results in getting different types of fat having different melting points that would ultimately affect the crystalline structure of fat in cream and thereby the resultant butter. In order to have better control different processes are available that may be followed depending on season and type of fat. Some of these methods are described here under.

A. ***Cold/warm/cold ripening*** : Cream is rapidly cooled at 5°C and held for 2-3 hours. During warm phase the temperature selected should be 1°-2°C below the melting point of fat so that the shell forming triglycerides remain in crystalline form. During second cooling phase the temperature is kept at 8°-12°C and the cream is held at this temperature for 12-15 hours in order to stabilize the crystalline fat fraction.

B. ***Warm /cold /cold ripening*** : This system is mainly suited for soft fat. Here the cream after pasteurization is first cooled to 21°-23°C to initiate crystallization of higher melting fat triglycerides. After 2-3 hours it is chilled to 6°C and held for another 2-3 hours. The temperature is then raised to 13°-14°C at which the cream is stored for 14-16 hours.

C. ***Warm ripening*** : Here the cream after pasteurization is cooled to 18°-21°C and held for 4-6 hours. This is also best suited for starter culture addition leading to diacetyl flavour development.

D. ***Cold ripening*** : Here the cream after pasteurization is cooled to 13°-16°C and held for 16-22 hours.

For firm butter : Cool cream at constant temperature (13°/13°/13°C)

For softer butter : Cool cream in steps which will result in less solid fat, larger fat crystals and greater proportion of solid fat inside fat globules. To achieve this "ALNARP" method is followed for cream ageing/ripening where temperature is controlled as follows – (8°/20°/14°C).

Addition of Colour

The aesthetic quality of food is judged with first sensory quality that is colour. Foods that are pleasing to eyes are more likely to be consumed, thereby contributing varied diets and better nutrition. Both synthetic and natural food colours, therefore, play a significant role in making the acceptable processed food products during manufacture, storage and quality control. Colours also supplement natural appearance of processed foods to ensure batch-to-batch uniformity when raw materials are available of varying intensities. To provide a even colour to butter through out the year irrespective of changes in the carotene content of milk fat due to seasonal effect and also where buffalo milk cream is used for butter making, natural or coal tar colouring matters may be used. This has a special significance in table butter manufacture.

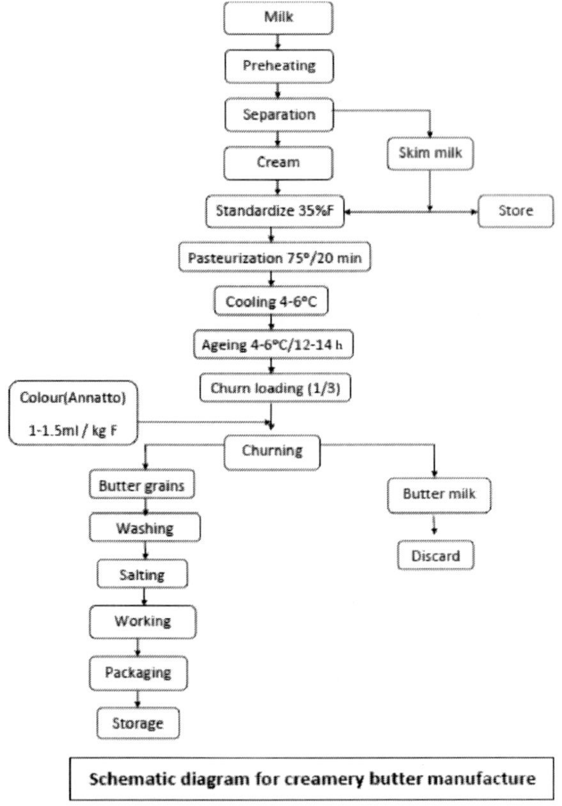

Schematic diagram for creamery butter manufacture

Natural butter colour may be obtained from vegetable sources like – vegetable oil extract from the seeds of "annatto" tree called "Bixa Oreliana". Annatto extracts are prepared by leaching the seeds with one or more of approved food grade solvents such as edible vegetable oils and fats and alkaline and alcoholic solution. Depending on end use, the pigments from alkaline extracts are precipitated with food grade acids and further purified by re-crystallization from approved solvents. The major colouring compound of the oil soluble extract is carotenoid, bixin which shows fairly good light and heat stability but is susceptible to oxidation which is accelerated by heat and light. Bixin is primarily used in dairy and fat-based products such as processed cheese, butter, margarine. The seeds of annatto tree contains two shades of colour namely yellow and red as a thin coating. These colours are extracted from the seeds using a source of vegetable oil. Another source of butter colour is from the vegetable β-Carotene. It is isomer of naturally occurring carotenoid pigment, carotene. Carotene or provitamin A occurs naturally in products such as butter, cheese, carrots, alfalfa and yellow coloured cereal grains. β-carotene is sensitive to alkali and is very sensitive to air and light, especially at high temperatures. It is insoluble in water, ethanol, glycerine and propylene glycol but it slightly soluble in edible oils at room temperature. Unlike other natural identical carotenoid colourants allowed for food use, the FDA permits the addition of β-carotene to colour foods at any levels consistent with good manufacturing practices. It imparts a yellow - to orange colour at 2-500 ppm levels in foods. β-carotene is used to colour a wide range of foods such as butter, margarine. Carrot containing carotene which may also be used as a colouring matter for butter. Carrot is first micro-pulverized into a semi solid suspension then β-carotene is extracted using vegetable or butter oil in which it is soluble. Such a suspension contains about 500,000 units of vitamin A activity per gram.

The usual rate of addition is 1-2 ml of the concentrated colour extract per kg of fat present in the cream

Churning of Cream

Churning of cream consist of agitation at a suitable temperature until the fat globules adhere into larger mass or until complete separation of fat and serum occurs. In most cases it is achieved by beating-in of air in the churn partially filled with cream and rotating at several revolutions per minutes. The churning should proceed rapidly and completely and the formed butter grains should have the correct firmness to allow for efficient working. The ideal butter grain size is about the size of pea.

The major objective of churning is to produce butter.

In cream fat exist in the form of stable emulsion and in form of continuous phase. If it remains intact, butter can not be made. The emulsion has to be broken, to release fat from fat globules, by way of vigorous agitation.

Churning Process

Upon agitation great extension of air-plasma interface occur through incorporation of air bubbles. As soon as the fat globules comes in contact with the interface a part of membrane is spread out there along with liquid fat fraction. A belt of liquid fat remains attached with the fat globule that also retains part of its membrane. Fat globules are crowded on the interface and contact each other to form clumps. The liquid fat serves to cement these globules together through capillary cohesion forces. Another part of liquid fat forms a layer on the bubble surface inter-spread with very minute fat patches. Such a layer acts as foam dipressant causing it to burst. The fat layer on the surface of the bubble is then dispersed as particles of colloidal size in the plasma. On repeated formation and destruction of air bubbles the clumps grow into butter granules that contains more than 80% fat in the form of globules. This may be put forth as follows:

1. The fat globules touches air bubbles.
2. This spreads membrane substance and liquid fat over air-water interface and attach to the bubbles.
3. Air bubbles keeps moving and collide with each other and coalesce.
4. The adhering fat globules are driven towards each other.
5. Liquid fat acts as sticking agent and fat globules are clumped together.
6. Finally small fat clumps or butter grains are formed.

Alternatively we can say that when the cream is agitated a foam of large protein bubbles are formed. The membranes of fat globules, being surface active, are drawn towards the air-water interface and fat globules are concentrated in the foam. As agitation continues, the bubble becomes smaller, making the foam compact and thereby applying pressure on the fat globules. This results in partial disintegration of membrane and release of some part of liquid fat. The liquid fat containing fat crystals, spreads into a thin layer on the surface and on fat globules. As the bubble becomes more dense, the foam becomes unstable and more liquid fat is released. The fat globules combine into fine grains of butter that progressively grow larger as the process continues.

Theories of Churning

1. ***Phase reversal theory*** : This theory has been coined by Fisher and Hook. It postulates that agitation of cream during churning causes coalescence and clumping of fat globules until the ratio of surface area to volume of fat becomes so small that it no longer holds butter-milk in stable form. The oil-in-water emulsion suddenly breaks yielding butter grains (water-in-oil emulsion) and free butter-milk.

   However, this does not hold good because butter is not true water-in-oil emulsion and is found to contain intact fat globules as revealed during structural studies.

2. ***Foam theory*** : This theory was postulated by Rahn. According to this theory, the presence of foam is a must for churning. There exist a foam producing substance in cream which gradually solidifies during agitation. The fat globules tend to concentrate and clump on the foam bubble due to surface tension effect. The foam producing substance assumes a solid character and the foam collapses. The fat globules then coalesce and butter is formed.

   The theory fails on the ground that foam formation is not required in case of continuous butter making process.

3. ***Modern theory*** : This theory was given by King. It postulates the following:

   (i) In cooled cream the fat exist as clusters of fat globules within which the fat is present in partially solid and partially liquid form.

   (ii) Churning breaks clusters and causes foam formation. The globules concentrate in film around air bubbles and comes into close contact with each other.

   (iii) The direct concussion between globules causes gradual arosion of emulsion protecting surface layer (phospholipids and proteins). The globules then adhere to form large particles (butter grains).

   (iv) The globules under pressure yields enough free liquid fat during working to enclose water droplets, air bubbles and intact fat globules.

The theory seems to cover all aspects of butter making.

Factors Affecting Churnability of Cream

1. ***Fat percentage of cream*** : For an exhaustive churning the fat percent in the cream intended for butter making needs to be standardized. The process also helps in controlling the fat loss in butter-milk. To minimize fat loss, it is advisable to keep the optimum fat in cream between 30-35% with an average of 33%. An higher fat percentage in cream may result in shorter churning time and incomplete churning process leading to higher fat losses in butter-milk.

2. ***Fat composition of cream*** : Milk fat is a mixture of glycerides of widely varying melting and solidifying points. Low melting point fats are called soft fats and high melting points fats are called hard fats. An increased proportion of soft fats result in shorter churning time, increased fat loss and softer butter and visa-versa.

3. ***Fat globule size*** : cream containing smaller fat globules churn with difficulty. Higher proportion of small size fat globules result in longer churning time and greater fat loss in butter-milk. Smaller size of fat globules generally scapes churning action and pass into butter-milk. On the other hand large size fat globules containing more liquid fat tends to clump together more easily and are churned exhaustively thereby reducing fat loss.

4. ***Temperature of cream*** : This is also called churning temperature and is important in controlling rapidity and exhaustiveness of churning. The optimum churning temperature ranges from 9°-11°C. There is always a certain rise in temperature of cream during the churning process. An initial higher temperature of cream may result in shorter churning time, higher fat loss in butter-milk and weaker butter.

5. ***Churn load*** : All butter churns have certain total capacity. However, if they are filled completely there may not be enough space left to bring about agitation that is necessary to break the emulsion. It is therefore, advised that the churn may be filled upto 40% of its capacity (optimum ½ or $^{1}/_{3}$rd of total capacity). Both over and under loading may not give optimum result. Under loading may result in poor agitation, insufficient churning, rapid rise in temperature and difficulty in compositional control. Whereas, over loading may result in prolonged churning time, loss of fat in butter-milk, inferior body and texture of resultant butter and uneven colour of butter due to un-satisfactory working.

6. ***Speed of churning*** : Generally the manufacturer of butter churn advise an optimum speeds related to process of churning and working in order to get complete churning (to avoid fat excessive loss) and better working of butter (for even distribution of salt and water through out the body of butter). Optimally it takes about 70-80 revolutions for proper churning. An higher speed creates centrifugal force with no agitation to cream and breaking of emulsion.

The slow churning of cream : this refers to too long a churning time than the usual 35-40 minutes in case of cream having normal fat and right temperature of churning. It may be because of - too low temperature of the cream, over loading of churn, too high viscosity of cream which may be due to high fat content in cream or lipase action causing the cream to become ropy or it could be due to excessively low fat cream.

Over churning : this refers to condition where the churn is run for over time missing the exact break point of the emulsion. It may result in – un-satisfactory washing of butter grains that may enclose excessive butter-milk, coarse flavour of butter, defective body and texture of butter causing it to become leaky and greasy, low keeping quality of butter and difficulty in controlling the composition of butter.

Excessive fat loss in buttermilk may be caused due to – too short churning time allowing scape of too small fat globules and butter grains to pass in butter-milk, too low or too high fat content in cream, improper neutralization and pasteurization of cream, excessive agitation during cooling and no holding of cooled cream, partial churning during pumping of cream, high churning temperature, over loading of churn and too high speed of churning.

Butter Churns

A butter churn is basically a container used to bring about agitation of cream to eventually form butter. The main purpose of the churn is to agitate cream so that the emulsion is broken and the phase inversion takes place to obtain fine grains of butter fat. The grains are then washed to remove excess butter-milk and are worked to form a compact mass called butter. There are several , designs and shapes of butter churn available. The earlier butter churns both, hand and power operated were made up of wood. The modern butter churns are made of steel and are mostly power operated with arrangements for controlling speed for different operations during butter making. Different types may be classified as follows

1. ***Dash churns*** : These churns have stationary cream holding vessel whereas agitators and dashers are provided in the form of plunger, disc or blades which are movable. The movement of dashers brings about agitation of cream inside the vessel in order to break the emulsion.

2. ***Swinging churns*** : Here the vessel is made to move forward and backwards in a horizontal plane. The vessel has internal diaphragms of longitudinal or diagonal sections for intensive agitation of cream.

3. ***Rotary churns*** : These are mostly barrel type having many shapes like cylindrical, conical, cubical and tetrahedral with adjustable speeds and fitted with axial strips and dashers.

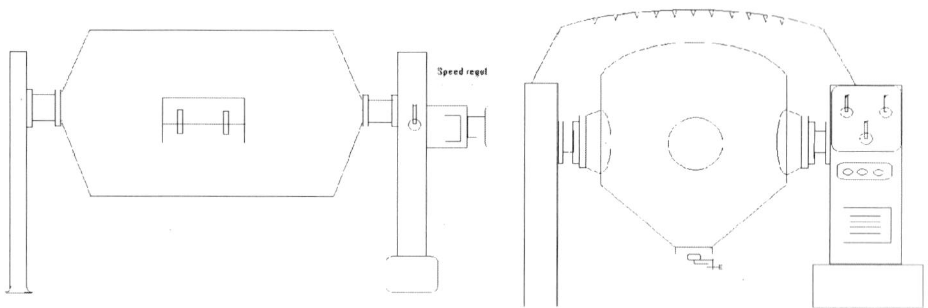

Fig. 4.3: Cylindrical churn

Fig. 4.4: Conical churn

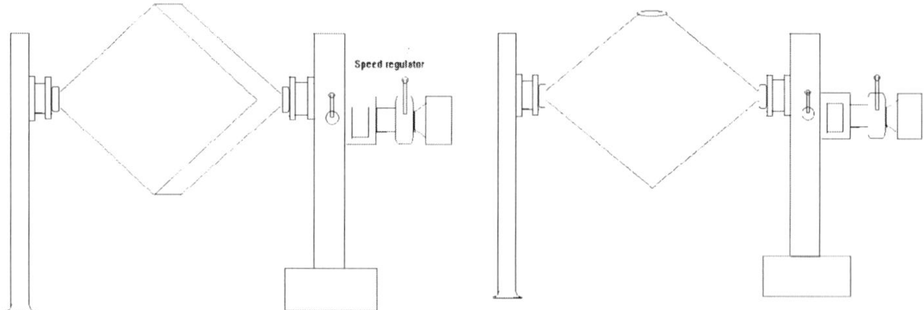

Fig. 4.5: Cubical churn

Fig. 4.6: Double cone churn

The above designs of churns generally have capacities ranging from 1000-15000 Kgs. If filled 40% of their capacity are capable of churning cream at 8°-10°C within 30-45 minutes (max. 50 min.) with a fat recovery of 99.5-99.7% and fat loss of less than 1% in butter-milk.

Draining of Buttermilk

The process of butter making is to agitate the cream to bring about phase inversion from oil-in-water emulsion to water-in-oil type emulsion. The point at which the change in emulsion phase takes place is called the break point. As soon as the break point is reached the butter grains are separated form the serum which is then called butter-milk. It is important to remove this butter milk before more of it is enclosed in the butter grains. Therefore, just after break point is reached, the butter-milk is allowed to drain through a strainer to avoid losing butter grains in serum. However, some of the butter milk remains entrapped between the grains. This may be removed by subsequent operations.

Washing of Butter Grains

In this operation butter grains are mixed with portable water in an amount equal to the amount of butter-milk removed. The main purpose of washing is:

a. To remove loose butter-milk from butter grains,

b. To reduce the curd content of butter,

c. To obtain butter of correct firmness,

d. To decrease intensity of off-flavours and

e. To improve the quality of butter made.

It is advisable to use freshly pasteurized and cooled water which is chemically and microbiologically safe. This is important specially in case of table butter manufacture. The temperature of wash water used should be 1°-2°C lower than the churning temperature of cream. This helps to maintain firmness of butter. After addition of wash water the churn is closed and allowed to have few revolutions before the wash water is drained out. If need be another washing may be given to the grains to completely remove the loose butter-milk thereby reducing the curd content of the butter and to have better compositional control.

Salting of Butter

Salt is added to the table butter to preserve it against microbes and to add to the taste as butter is usually used as a spread on bread. Salt is added at the rate of 2-2.5% of the butter out turn (expected yield). It may be added as dry salt by way of sprinkling or in the form of 12% brine solution. The most suitable level of salt for most customers appears to be 2.3%. Over salting may result in coarse texture and briny flavour in butter. The major objectives are:-

a. To season butter for high palatability

b. To aid in preventing growth of bacteria, yeast and mould

c. To increase the over-run

The salt should be evenly distributed through out the mass of butter. Uneven distribution of salt may result in compositional differences, leaky texture, wavy colour and grittiness which is caused due to addition of dry salt to very soft butter or low moisture butter, using salt that has low solubility. Control of salt involves – correct determination of amount of fat present, correct calculation of amount of salt to be added, correct weighing of dry salt and proper distribution/incorporation with butter granules.

Salt for addition to butter should have following characteristics:

1. Contains high percentage (99%) of sodium chloride.
2. It should be free from bitter tasting compounds.
3. It should have low moisture content.
4. Should quickly dissolve in water resulting in clear brine.
5. It should be free from bacteria and mould.
6. It should be free from extraneous matter.

Working of Butter

This refer to kneading of butter granules and rendering them into continuous mass. The objectives of working are as follows –

1. To expel butter-milk.
2. To regulate moisture content in butter.
3. To completely dissolve and properly incorporate the salt.
4. To bring butter grains into a compact mass.
5. To reduce moisture droplets to microscopic size.

This can be achieved by squeezing butter through perforated plates (continuous machine), squeezing through rollers as in hand butter worker or by allowing to fall from a height as in case of modern butter churns. Working helps to closely knit the butter grains into tough waxy texture and even distribution of salt and moisture. Working increases the air content of butter in the form of fine bubbles.

Normally butter contains 0.5-10 ml air per 100g of butter with an average of 4 ml/ 100g. Under working produces leaky butter having free moisture on the surface of butter. This may lead to lower keeping quality and may attract bacteria and mould during storage. Whereas, excessive or over working may damage body and texture of butter.

Working of butter may also be done under vaccum (0-68 cm Hg). This would result in denser butter with more glossy appearance and close texture.

Moisture control in butter is done to meet the legal standards and get over run for maximum profit. Before butter is drawn from the churn the moisture content is determined in order to make sure it does not contain lower or higher moisture than desired. If need be, the amount of water to be added can be calculated using the following formula:-

Amount of water to be added = (Final moisture required – first moisture test)/ 100 x amount of butter in the churn.

Once the amount of water is calculated, clean portable and pasteurized and cooled water is added directly to the churn and it is further worked to evenly distribute the moisture droplets throughout the body of butter. No loose water droplets should be visible on the body of the butter.

Over Run in Butter

It is the increase in the amount of butter made form the given amount of fat in the cream. It is caused by the presence of salt, moisture and curd. It is expressed

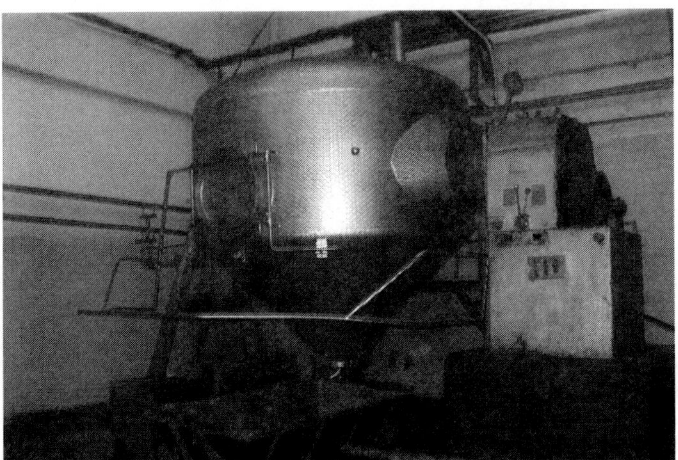

Fig. 4.7: Factory butter churn

in terms of percentage. It is a source of profit for butter maker and helps check the efficiency of operations. Theoretically, as per legal standard butter should contain 80% fat. Starting from 100 kg fat, maximum amount of butter that can be made is (100/80) x 100 = 125 kg. Meaning that maximum over run obtainable, theoretically is around 25%. However, in practice this is never achieved. An average of 20-22% of over run may be achieved under best controlled conditions. The formula for calculating the over run is as follows:-

Percent over run (% OR) = (B – F/F) x 100

Where, B is the amount of butter made (kg) and F is the amount of fat in churn (kg)

Yield of Butter

This means the total amount of butter obtained from total amount of fat in cream. Normally it should be about 79-85%. The yield of butter can be calculated using the formula:–

Yield (Y) = F x (100 + % over run)/100

Where, Y is the yield of butter in kg and F is amount of fat in cream in kg.

Butter Making Processes

A. ***Batch process*** : To manufacture butter of uniform colour throughout the year, cream is coloured artificially by adding butter colour (annatto). The quantity of colour to be added depends whether cream from cow or buffalo is being used. The cream is churned at 10°C to obtain butter of firm consistency. The loss of fat in butter-milk does not exceed 0.2 percent. The process of churning should not exceed 30 to 40 minutes. When the cream is churned into butter and the butter milk serum becomes clear, water at 3° to 4°C lower than the churning temperature is added, and the churning continued till butter granules are of the size of white kernels. Butter-milk is drawn off at this stage and the butter is washed two or three times with fresh clean water. Adequate quantity of salt is then added and the butter is worked so that the salt is uniformly incorporated, and it does not contain any excess moisture. The butter is then packed for marketing. Table butter should contain not less than 80 percent milk fat and not more than 16 percent moisture. It may contain upto 2 percent salt and may be coloured with annatto. No preservative is permissible. Diacetyl may be added to the extent of 4 ppm to impart flavour to butter.

B. ***Continuous butter making*** : Until 1937 butter was being made in small lots by way of churning the cream using butter churn of different shape, size and designs. The first continuous butter making was developed in 1940 based on Fritz principle and quickly gained wide acceptance in countries manufacturing un-salted or lightly salted butter. However, it was not until late 1960 that satisfactory salting method was developed for continuous butter making process. Soon the batch churning process was replaced with continuous process in all major butter producing countries. The existing continuous butter making machines developed during and after World war II, can be classify, broadly into three basic groups/principles/processes.

1. ***Churning process*** : This process involves churning of cream of normal composition , using high speed beaters to break the fat emulsion in chilled cream and cause formation of butter grains, in a matter of seconds. The butter-milk is allowed to drain followed by salting and working before the product is extruded form the machine in the shape of ribbon. This is the most common process and machine based on this principle includes - Fritz process (Germany), Westfalia (Sweden) and Silkeborg (Denmark).

2. ***Concentration and phase reversal process*** : In this process first the normal cream containing 30-40% fat is re-separated to produce cream having 80-82% fat in a special cream separator. The concentrated cream which is now called "butter mix" is subjected to cooling and mechanical agitation to cause phase reversal and thus converted into butter before expulsion from the machine. The machines based on this principle includes – New way process (Australia), Alfa process (German) and Alfa Laval process (Sweden).

3. ***Emulsification process*** : Here also the normal cream is re-separated to get 87-94% fat. The butter mix thus obtained is passed through a chiller followed by texturator, in order to completely crystallize the fat. The contents are then worked by bpassing through the perforated discs and the butter emerges through the opening directly to a packaging machine. The machines based on this principle includes – Cherry Barrel (USA) and Kraft (USA).

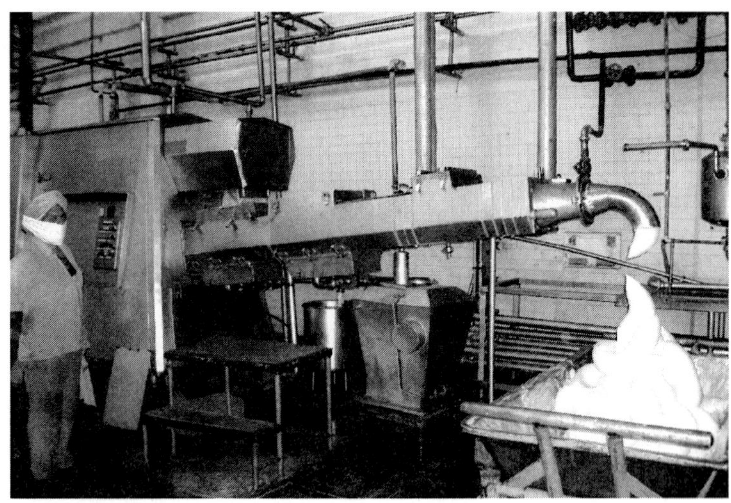

Fig. 4.8: Continuous butter making machine

Butter manufacture using continuous machine offers following advantages:-

a. Greater control over manufacturing process.
b. Greater uniformity of body and texture of finished product.
c. Better salt and moisture distribution.
d. More hygienic process-free from contamination, being closed system.
e. Requires less space and labour
f. Lower processing cost-ecomomical
g. Quicker process-time required is around 5-7 minutes.
h. Higher capacity plant-500-2000 kg/hour.

A number of different systems have now been developed for regular commercial use. The advantages of continuous system includes, less economy in capital and running cost, no time loss for fat crystallization, less wastage, hygienic being closed system free from air borne contamination.

Fritz process

The milk is pumped from the receiving vats to a separator from which cream of 40-50 percent is obtained. The cream is pasteurized to 95°C without holding, cooled to 6-10°C and held for some hours (or overnight) in a storage vat tank. Next, it is pumped into a small control container which maintains the flow of cream at a constant pressure and adjustable rate. The cream is then passed into a small water-jacketed cylinder (about 25cm. Long and 25cm. in diameter) which is kept cool by circulating cold water in the jacket. High-speed vanes in this cylinder churn the cream into butter in 1-2 seconds. The buttermilk and butter granules drop into an inclined section fitted with 2 spiral screws about 45cm long and 15 cm in diameter, which rotate in opposite directions. Here the buttermilk runs off and butter is forced through a perforated plate from the farther side of which it is removed by rotating blades. It emerges as a ribbon 7.5 cm x 3.7 cm in cross section, which can be bulk packed directly or cut and wrapped into retail sized pats.

Alfa-laval process

The milk is preheated to 45-50°C (113-122°F) and passed on to a hermetic Alfa-Laval separator to produce cream with a 25-35 percent fat content. This cream is then pasteurized at 95°C and passed in a special cream separator to the fat content desired in the butter. In a small standardizing vat/tank, the calculated amount of salt, water or skim milk can be added to allow for the adjustment of the composition of butter. The plastic cream is then pumped through the transmutator where it changes from cream to butter. The transmutator consists of three jacketed stainless steel cylinder (each about 180cm long and 30cm. In diameter) inside each of which rotates a stainless steel drum fitted with raised spiral strips. Brine circulates in the jackets at variable temperatures. Phase inversion starts in the first cylinder and is actually completed in the second one. The butter leaves the third cylinder in a semi-fluid form and is packaged immediately. Solidification takes places at once and is completed in the cold store.

Cherry burrell's process

The cream is pumped from the receiving vats, through an agitating heater to destabilize the emulsion, and then directly to the centrifugal separator which concentrates the cream upto 86-90 percent fat, and breaks the emulsion. An automatic desludging type separator is used. Next, the butterfat containing dispersed serum is pasteurized in a vacreator, cooled to 43-46°C and passed into standardizing vats. The standardization of acidity, moisture and salt content is an intermittent process. After standardization, the butter mix is pumped through a chiller resembling an ice cream freezer and cooled to 5°C. It then passes through a texturator which crystallizes the fat more completely and later works the butter slightly by making it flow through a perforated plate.

The butter emerges through a mouth-piece into a packing machine or bulk container. The whole process takes about half an hour.

Manufacturing Process

The preparation of cream is done in the same way as for conventional churning before it is fed, continuously, from the ripening/ ageing tank to the continuous butter making machine. In general continuous butter making machine consists of four different sections namely:

Churning cylinder : This section consist of horizontal cylinder equipped with a double cooling and multi speed agitator/beater. The distance between the cylinder wall and the beater is only few milli-meters. The beater speed ranges from 0-1400 rpm. The cream from the aging tank is fed to the churning cylinder via a balance tank by means of a positive displacement pump, to the rear of the churning section. To ensure proper churning, proper flow rate control is essential. A rapid conversion takes place in the cylinder with a resident time of 1-2 seconds. The grains and the butter-milk then pass to another section.

Separation section : After the fat emulsion is broken in the churning cylinder, the butter grains and the butter-milk together enter this section. The separation section is equipped with a screw conveyer (augers) and is inclined. The necessary perforated plates are fitted at the back of inclined tube to facilitate drainage of butter milk. Wash water is also introduced at this stage for washing of butter grains and adjust their size to enable efficient drainage of butter-milk. At the end of this section ,there are series of perforated plates and mixing vanes followed by a flow regulating gate. The speed of auger and degree of opening of this gate will effect back pressure on the butter and thus effect drainage of butter-milk. The butter grains are carried forward by the screw conveyer to the next section.

Squeeze –drying section (first working) : As the butter grains leaves the separation section , they pass through a conical channel and a perforated plate to the squeeze drying section where any remaining butter milk is removed. A 50/50 slurry of salt and water is injected using a high pressure injector, between the first and second working plates in this section. Salt solution may also be injected in the first chamber of second working section in some machines. To have correct quantity of salt in butter, a positive pump is used for accurate dozing of salt solution. The salt used should be finally ground having 40-48 nm particle size and the concentration should not exceed 55% in the slurry.

The slurry to be prepared 30 minutes before churning begins and should be agitated vigorously. Every endeavour is made to distribute salt as completely as possible within the short time while the butter is passing through the working discs/plates. The lumps of butter then proceed to another section of the machine.

Second working section : This section works under vacuum and consist of four small sub-sections which are separated from the adjacent one by a perforated plate. Perforated plates of different sizes and working impellers of different shapes are used to optimize treatment of the butter. In the first small sub-section pasteurized and cooled portable water is injected for final adjustment of moisture content. The butter passes through a series of perforated plates. The finished butter is discharged from the end nozzle as a continuous ribbon into butter silo and then pumped to the packaging machine or directly into the well synchronized packaging machine. Transmitters for moisture content, salt content, density and temperature can be fitted in the outlet for monitering the process. Measuring the dielectrical constant of butter, the moisture percentage can be measured and consequently adjusted to the desired level. The entire system of manufacturing can be computer controlled with continuous digital readout of the functions of separate components.

Packaging of Butter

The butter is generally stored in a packaged form. As soon as the butter is produced it is bulk packed into 25-40 kg boxes or tubs lined with parchment paper / butter paper and stored at – 22° C to – 29° C for 24 – 48 hours before it is packed into smaller packs or chiplets for retail marketing. The objectives of good packaging are:-

1. To offer protection against contamination and damage.
2. To protect against loss of moisture that may lead to weight loss.
3. To protect against flavour deterioration.
4. For easy and safe transportation.

For retail purpose butter is packed in 25, 50, 100, 250 and 500 gram packing. Larger pack of 250 and 500 g size are generally well rapped in parchment paper, for local consumption and for longer transportation into food grade plastic (poly-propylene) or laquared tin containers which are sealed with aluminium foil and covered with snap-on plastic lids. Smaller packs of 25, 50 and 100 g are first rapped into parchment paper and then placed into cardboard or paper board cartoons. 20-50 such small packs are then placed into bigger corrugated cardboard box for easy handling, storage and transportation.

Butter may also be packed into single service pack of 10-15 g in the form of chiplets. These chiplets may either be packed with butter paper followed with aluminium foil, or polypropylene tubs sealed with aluminium foil with extended lip for easy opening. This is performed using automatic packaging machine which cuts, pack and sealed each chiplet / tub. Each packed chiplet or tub are then placed into cardboard cartoon that holds 10-20 or more chiplets or tubs for easy shipment.

The technique involved in packing butter could be manual packing which is labour intensive and costly or it could be done mechanically. For this, fully automatic packaging units are available which mechanically moulds patts and wrap the product. At the end of packaging line the smaller packs (100g) are manually placed into cardboard cartoons designed to hold 20-50 or even more of such packs for ease of storage and transportation.

The machine can be reset for different size of mould patts. This is suitable for large scale operations and helps to reduce labour and cost of packaging and handling losses. Some of the well known brands of such packaging machines are – Kustner, Benhill (German), SIG (Swiss). The butter packed in boxes or cartoons is transferred to cold store (5° C) for a period of 24-48 hours and is then shifted to low temperature storage (- 25° C) until ready for transportation and usage.

Storage of Butter

As butter is a parishable product it should not be stored longer than necessary. However, when production exceed demand and to level out the fluctuations between flush and lean season, it becomes un-avoidable and the butter produced needs to be stored. For short period butter can be stored at 4°C. However, in case the butter is to be stored for longer period, it is stored at temperatures ranging from -23° to -29°C. Only best quality butter should be stored for longer period.

Usage of Butter

Butter is generally used as yellow fat spread for direct table consumption. However, being the concentrated source of milk fat it may be used for standardization of various dairy products like ice-cream, reconstituted milk etc. Un-salted butter may be converted into products like butter oil and ghee. Butter is successfully used in cooking of several dishes and is widely used in the confectionary industry for preparation of cakes, pastries, cookies etc.

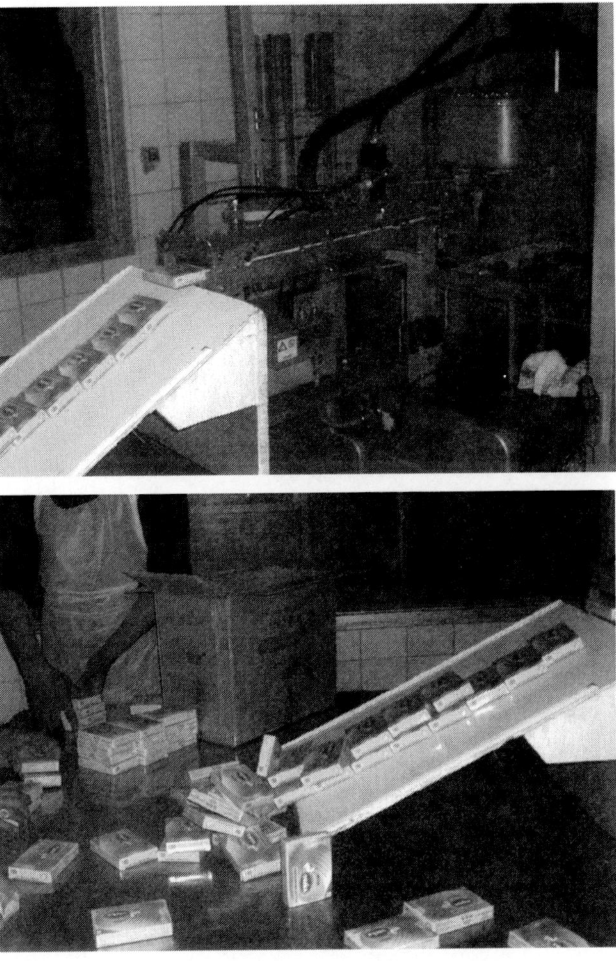

Fig. 4.9: Butter packaging machine

Special Butters

1. Whipped butter is regular butter whipped for easier spreading. Whipping increases the amount of air in butter and increases the volume of butter per pound. For the production of whipped butter, the butter is soften to 20-24°C, so that it is soft enough to work easily. At this stage colour and salt will be added, then product is whipped to get the desired over-run (50 to 100%), packed and stored at refrigerated temperature. It may contain butter fat around 45 to 50%, so its caloric value is less than that of butter.

2. Whey Butter is butter made from whey separated from curd during the making of cheese. It is a strong tasting with a bit of a cheesy flavour in it. It can be salty tasting, if salt was added to the cheese-making process

before the whey was drained off. It will be less shiny than regular butter and a deeper yellow. It may have added salt and annatto colouring, just as regular butter would. It may contain residual starter cultures from the cheese batch, and added casein.

Whey cream will be prepared from three sources of whey, particularly cheese, paneer and chhana. The fat content of the cream should range from 40 to 45 percent. The cream should be smooth and free from lumps. After separation of cream, it should be cooled to 4-7°C. Then cream should be heat treated/pasteurized at 60° C for 20 minutes or at 85° C for 15 seconds. Vacreation method/plate heat exchanger can be used for pasteurization and cool quickly to 4°C.

The butterfat content will end up being between 80 and 90%. In Canada, the legal definition is that it must be a minimum of 80% butterfat by weight. In Ireland, it will be 82% butterfat, 16% water, and 2% milk solids.

It is popular in Sweden, where it is sold in most stores as an everyday butter called "mess-smor". In other parts of the world, Whey Butter is used commercially in baked goods and in making candies. Whey butter had the softest texture compare to regular butter.

3. Flavoured Butter is popular in western world to use in sandwiches and spreads. Flavourings are added to enhance the taste of the product. Natural flavourings such as dry onion powder, chilly powder, pepper powder and ginger powder can be used. These were mixed after butter is prepared and care should be taken to minimize the contamination as these ingredients are added directly to butter after butter being made.

Structure of Butter

Milk and cream are natural emulsions consisting of a dispersed phase of fat in a liquid continuous phase. To considerable extent the fat globules are stabilized by phospholipids and to some extent by casein, albumin and globulin. In contrast Butter and Oleomargarine are emulsions of water in oil with a plastic continuous phase. They contain 80% fat and the remainder consists of salt, proteins and water. Stability of butter and Margarin is maintained by semi solid consistency of continuous phase rather than by perfect emulsification. The original cream is the suspension of fat globules in an emulsion of casein in an aqueous solution of lactose. The fat globules are coated with a membrane that consists of an incomplete layer of lipoprotein. When the cream is agitated the fat globules are denuded of the membrane surrounding them and are free to coalesce. Some of the original fat globules may survive the process – considerably in some continuous process. Much of the fat remains in globular form though the globules have been stripped of their membrane and appears to retain their identity and having at their surface a monomolecular layer of crystalline fat. The fat globules in cream having sufficient stability to withstand shear forces of churning process are those with 0.1-0.5 μm thick shell of solid fat and with small crystalline aggregates of varying size and shape of liquid fat in the interior. Consequently the amount of globular fat present in butter depends on the mechanical treatment during the manufacturing process.

Although the amount of globular fat falls rapidly with increasing working intensity still 26-35% of the total fat content is present in globular form. Numerous electron microscopy pictures have distinguished between two typical structures, a globular or grain structure and an almost completely homogenous structure caused by mechanical working. A strong correlation between type of structure and the consistency of butter exist with increasing homogeneity.

During the churning process the oil in water emulsion is transformed into a water in oil emulsion. During the process the fat globule membrane is damaged and liquid fat is squeezed out of the globules causing them to clump so that the emulsion is broken and phase inversion occurs. After the churning process the fat becomes the continuous phase and water the dispersed phase. The fat phase in butter made either by traditional or continuous process, is not a homogenous phase. There are present two different fat phases in butter, namely a continuous phase of free fat and dispersed in this is a globular phase consisting of relatively intact fat globules. At the same time the interfacial tension forces between the serum and the hydrophobic fat are such that they cause the serum to break up into small droplets, which vary in diameter from 1-10 μm.

Butterfat consists of a mixture of saturated and unsaturated glycerides of the fatty acids. At the temperature at which the butter is churned much of the fat is solid. It is the characteristic of the glycerides that when they are cooled they do not crystallize immediately. If the temperature is just below the melting point little or no crystallization may take place. The crystals develop around the nucleation point. Once the nucleus is formed they tend to persist in the fat because little movement is possible in the highly viscose melt. The glyceride molecules are elongated, so that the characteristic crystal formation is needle like. But as the crystals grow these may amalgamate and form plates with a thickness of upto 20 μm.

As the cream is agitated, the crystals that already exist in the fat globules become disrupted and the fragments take up more or less random positions within the fat that eventually surrounds the newly formed water droplets. Such a network may have quite an open structure and yet have considerable rigidity. The remainder of the space between the globules will be filled with the still liquid fat. Buried within this fat are the remains of the casein and other material that was resident as a membrane on the fat globules. The rigidity of the fat phase is largely controlled by the proportion of fat that is solid and therefore it is able to form a matrix. The internal crystallization increases the rigidity of the globules, which scarcely influences consistency, but external crystallization in the continuous fat phase results in formation of solid network of fat crystals grown together, strongly influences the consistency. This results in considerable increase in firmness of butter. The number of crystal platelets, which generally have a parallel orientation, increases during storage of the butter.

The water provides arrears of weakness in the structure that may lead to incipient cracks when the butter is sheared. It is possible to include upto 25%, by volume, of water while still retaining the emulsion structure. More usually 15% of the total volume is water, in which the salt and other water-soluble components of original cream is dissolved. At this concentration the droplets are separated by distance commensurate by their mean diameter. In a well-made butter well over 99.9% of the water exist in this droplet form.

Fat in Butter

Fat occurs in butter, in two forms

(i) ***Globular form*** : which ranges from 8-30% with an average diameter of 3.8 μ and the number of globules are in order of 9 x 106 per cubic ml. the globules have a layer next to the membrane that has a thicknes of about 1/10 th of the fat globule and consist of crystal of higher melting point fats oriented radially to the surface of globules. The center of the fat globule is occupied by liquid fat. This lends rigidity to the fat globules.

(ii) ***Free fat form*** : This occurs in two ways – (a) By squeezing portion of fat from globules during churning and (b) Through smashing fat globules during working of butter.

In both forms part of fat is liquid and part crystalline. The ratio of liquid to crystalline fat depends on (a) milk fat composition, (b) manufacturing technique and (c) temperature of butter making. Liquid fat constitutes fat phase of the butter. The amount of liquid fat is associated with spreadability. The crystalline fat constitute part of dispersed fat phase and includes crystals of lower melting point TG. The crystal size ranges from 0.1 micron to several hundred microns. The crystals exist in number of forms and are determined by the angle of tilt. Rapid and deep cooling produces gamma crystals consisting of low & high melting TG, whereas slow cooling produces beta crystals consisting of only high melting point TG, which are unstable. The structure of crystalline portion of fat plays an important role in the physical properties of butter. The size, shape, quantity and mutual arrangements of individual fat crystals are important elements of the crystal structure. Continuous butter making method, where fat is rapidly cooled with no globules and crystal size of 30-40 μ, have remarkebly different crystal structure and have different physical properties as compared to conventionally churned butter having many globules with fat crystals arranged at periphery.

The fat crystal size is undoubtedly an important factor. When pure fat is cooled rapidly very small crystals with maximum diameter of 1-2 μ are formed. Where as, slow cooling results in formation of large crystals with diameter upto 40 microns. The crystal formation proceeds from the center and reaches the size of upto 80-100 microns. Such crystals are structurally weak and break into irregular fragments upon slight agitation. Butter made from rapidly cooled cream contains more crystalline fat as a result of mixed crystal formation.

Table 4.7: Structural elements of butter

Element	Number (per ml) concentration	Proportion of butter (% vol/vol)	Dimension (μm)
Fat globules	10 x10	10-50	2.00-8.00
Fat crystals	10 x13	10-40	0.01-2.00
Moisture	10 x 10	13-15	1.00-25.00
Air cells	10 x 7	2-5	18.00-20.00

Source : Mulder & Walstra, 1974

Texture of Butter

This is essential to the quality of butter as it determines spreadability and effects appearance, taste, mouthfeel and suitability for many applications. Good quality butter should neither be too firm nor too soft and have sufficient standing property. It should be free from textural defects such as crumbly, gummy, sticky, greasy etc. Texture of butter is influenced by fat crystals of high melting triglycerides that form the three dimensional network and lends rigidity. The amount of crystalline fat and the size of individual crystal plays an important role in determining the strength of the structure. The crystal network is held together by reversible bonds (Vander Walls forces) which accounts for the coherence of the butter. When butter grains are worked (kneaded) together they form a mass of continuous network wherein fat globules, water globules and fat crystals are enclosed in addition to small volume of air. The firmness of butter is determined to the large extent by the proportion of solids in the fat. The nature and size of fat crystal may also affect the consistency of fats. The given proportion of crystals from heterogenous fat gives greater firmness than the same proportion of crystals from homogenous fat. Rapid cooling of fat results in smaller crystal size and high solid fat content. Both these factors favour high hardness and firmer butter. Slow cooling results in relatively low solid fat content and large crystals that favours low hardness and softer butter.

Renovation of Butter

Renovation means restoration, remodeling, improving. In case of butter, after butter fat gets rancid then that butter fat is treated to improve its acceptability after removing rancid odours by treatment. Thus renovated butter is butter which has become rancid and is then subjected to a process of renovation, by which the disagreeable odors and flavors are removed. It is not an unwholesome product, but should not be sold at butter prices. The butter is melted so as to draw off the brine for straining out the curd and other insoluble material, and then is deodorized by blowing air or steam through it. It is then cooled and churned with fresh cream, and is finally worked and packed for market like other butter.

Fractionation of Milk Fat

The physical properties such as melting point and consistency of butter are depending on chemical composition of the milk fat. The different triglycerides have different melting points and can therefore easily divided into different fractions consists of different fatty acids. When molten milk fat is slowly cooled, a crystalline solid and an un crystallized liquid phase are formed. Separation of these phases yields fractions with high and low softening points respectively. Fractional crystallization is most promising process to separate milk fat, a laboratory method of fractional crystallization is explained in detail in following paragraph.

Process

Milk fat was melted completely and washed several times with warm water, dried under vacuum and filtered at 50-60°C. 500g sample was melted in a beaker which is kept over thermostatically controlled water bath at 60°C. Fat was stirred at about 100 rpm. Then crystallization temperature was adjusted from 25°C to 32°C at an interval of 1°C for six hours. After crystallization at one of these temperatures fat was filtered on a Buchner funnel resulting in a liquid and a solid fraction at each of the selected temperatures. Fatty acid composition was determined using gas-liquid chromatographic determination.

Advantages/Applications of Fractionation

1. Spreadability of butter can be improved at refrigerated temperature by fractionating low melting point fatty acids from butter.
2. For the production of cocoa butter equivalents from palm oil and palmkernel oil can be made.
3. These fractions are useful in the study of milk composition and structure and also to determine the physiological effects when supplied with the diet.

Defects in Butter

Depending upon the type of cream, its age, acidity, cooling processing involved, packing and storage of butter various defect can appear into final product. Some common flavour, body-texture and colour defect are given here under

Table 4.8: Some common defects in butter

Flavour	Cause	Body & texture	Cause	Colour	Cause
Acidic/sour	High acid, under neutralized cream	Crumbly	Presence of hard fats, chilling just after making	Mottled	Inadequate washing & working
Neutralizer	Over neutralization	Greasy	Over working, high wash water temp.	Streaky/ wavy	Uneven working, incomplete working of 2 lots
Cooked	Over heating	Leaky	High churning temp., over churning, under working.	Dull/pale	Less colouring material, over working
Fishy	High acid salted butter, longer storage	Gritty	Incorrect salting, undissolved salt		
Rancid	Fat hydrolysis	Sticky	Over working		
Yeasty	Old cream				

Microbial Deterioration/Spoilage of Butter

Growth of micro organisms in butter causes a variety of color and flavour defects. Most of the MO's in cream gets killed during pasteurization, the spoilage organisms mainly come through post pasteurization steps and butter making. The defects in butter mainly attributed to the presence of psychotropic bacteria (lipolytic & proteolytic), yeast and molds. The psychotropic bacteria which are entering the product through unhygienic equipment grow during low temperature storage. However, molds create problems and relatively high temperature as prevalent India.

A. Color defects (Discoloration)

Discoloration of butter may be caused by bacteria, yeasts and molds. However major color defect in butter are caused by yeast and molds.

Bacterial Discoloration

a) ***Black discoloration (like grease smudge) causative organisms: Pseudomonas nigrificance:*** Due to butter stored @ low temperature (optimum for pigmentation is 4°C i.e. 15-20% salt concentration in the moisture droplets.

b) ***Fungal discoloration:*** Butter gets discolored due to surface growth of molds and the defect is also described as 'moldy butter'. This is a major defect commonly occurred in India since the ambient temperature storage condition encourages the growth of Fungi in butter. Fungi growth also favored by higher moisture content and acidity. Some psychotropic molds like Alternaria, Harmodendrum, phoma and stamphylium have been appear to grow in butter (unsalted) at low temperature (5°C) slight growth @-4 to -6°C but not @ -7 to -9°C. Some common fungal discoloration frequently occurred in butter are as follows -

Mould	Discoloration	Causative agent
	Black	Cladosporium harbarum, Aspergillus, Hasmodendrum, Alternaria, Mucor, Rhizopus, Staphylium
	Brown	*Aspergillus* spp, *Phoma* spp (muddy brown)
	Green & blue green	*Penicillium* spp., *Aspergillus* spp
	Orange & yellow	*Geotrichum candidum*
	Reddish pink	Fusarium
Yeast	Black	*Torula* spp
	Pink	*Rhodotorula* spp

B. Flavor defects

Rancid & putrid or cheesy odour is the most common flavor defects in butter. The other defects like malty, shunk-like flavor yeasty may also occur in butter.

a. ***Rancid flavor***: Butter gets rancid due to microbial, enzymatic or chemical degradation of fat constituents. The fat hydrolysis in butter mainly due to the activity of microbial lipases. Many of the lipolytic microorganisms are psychotropic and are able to grow at temperature slightly under 0°C and survive cold storage at -10°C. Some of the lipase producing organisms which can grow on butter is as follows.

Bacteria	Mould	Yeast
Ps. frage	Geotrichism Candidum	Candida lypolitica
P. fluoreseene	Cladosporium botyri	*Torulopsis* spp
P. putida	*Penicillium* spp	*Rhodotorula* spp
Achromobacter lipolyticum	*Aspergillus* spp	Sacharomyces fragilis

b. ***Putrifactor taint*** : This defect is due to breakdown of proteins by proteolytic enzymes produced by various organisms like *Pseudomonas putrefaciens, coliform, flavobacterium maloloris*. The chemical compound which is produced during the breakdown of protein is closely related to ovaleric acid which is responsible for off-flavor. The causative organism enter butter through un-chlorinated water supplies and equipments (butter churns, Cream vats)

c. ***Cheese taints*** : Cheese like flavors in butter is due to association action of different Gram negative rods shaped bacteria due to butter stored above 10°C.

Other flavor taints

i. ***Malty flavor*** : The formation of 3-methyl butanol in butter mainly responsible for malty flavor. It is due to the presence and growth of *Streptococcus lactis* variable *maltigenes* in cream.

ii. ***Shunk-like flavor*** : This defect is caused by - *Pseudomonas mephitica*

iii ***Fishy taint*** : Fishiness is developed due to decomposition of lecithin to trimethyl amine by microbes. The causative organism for fishiness are - *Pseudomonas ichthyosmia, Geotrichum candidum,* Yeasts.

Public Health Importance

Butter is not an ideal medium for the growth of pathogenic or food poisoning organisms due to high fat content, yet it may carry certain pathogen if contaminated during production, handling and packaging. Certain pathogens have been found to remain viable for long periods in butter. The possible sources of pathogens in butter may be the cream itself (improperly pasteurized) or the post-pasteurization contamination. Handler in the butter plant is usually the major sources of such organisms in butter.

Very few outbreaks of diseases or food poisoning have been reported so far from butter. *Staphylococys aureus* and salmonella have been encountered in butter.

Butter may, however, serves as a good medium for the growth molds including aflatoxins and other mycotoxins producers. Such toxins may cause serious health hazards in consumers. It is necessity to checking mold contamination and growth in butter.

Butter Powder

Butter with modification has been dried successfully. During production cream is separated to 62% fat and is homogenised in the presence of sodium citrate. High grade casein is dispersed in skim milk at 65-82°C. To the mixture is added sodium hydroxide, glycerol mono stearate (GMS) and permitted antioxidant and thoroughly mixed with cream solids, heated (70°C), spray dried, cooled and dry blended with free flowing agent (80% sodium aluminium silicate + 20% calcium phosphate). The product is bulk packed in fibre drum or vacuum packed retail containers with nitrogen to enhance shelf life (6 months). The typical composition is moisture 0.6%; fat 81.9%; S.n.f. 6.7%; emulsifier (GMS) 5.5%; Antioxidant 0.02% and caseinates 6.7%.

Suggested Readings

Arora, S. and Rai, T. (1997). Milk fat fractions: Properties and Applications. J. Dairying Food & Home Sci., 16:143-155.

Aneja, R.P., Mathur, B.N., Chandan, R.C. and Bannerjee, A.K. (2002). Fat rich products. In: Technology of Indian milk products. A Dairy India Publication.

De, S. (1980). Outlines of Dairy Technology. Oxford University Press, Delhi.

Edger Spree (1998). Milk and milk products technology. Marcel Dekker Inc., New York.

Freed, E. (2003). Butter – properties and analysis In: Encyclopaedia of Dairy Science, Vol 1, pp. 231.

Kinenai, M.P. (1986). Continuous Butter Manufacture. IDF Bulletin No.204:16-20.

Lambert, L.M. (1970). Modern Dairy Products. Chemical Publishing Co. Inc., New York.

McDowell, F.H. (1953). The Butter Makers Manual, New Zealand University Press.

Robinson, R.K. (1994). Modern Dairy Technology, Vol.I. Chapman and Hall, London.

5

Table Spreads

Introduction

The demand for butter as table spread has declined due to high cost, poor spreadability at low temperature, high saturated fat and cholesterol content, changing life style and increased demand for healthy products. Today food industry is actively involved in new product development, this includes new formulations and imitation of foods being designed to compete with or replace existing products based on their superiority in convenience, cost and quality. The wide acceptance of bread in regular diet among urban consumers (75 percent of all household) reflects around 8 percent rate of growth in bread consumption. With this increase, the requirement of a suitable spread to complement has also increased. Table spreads include a variety of spreadable semi-solid products such as fat spreads, cheese spread, peanut butter etc. Butter has also been blended with vegetable oils/fat to produce a product that retains dairy qualities of butter with enhanced spreadability. This was aimed towards maximizing flavour attributes of milk fat while utilizing the lubrication of liquid oil. Table spread is a water-in-oil type emulsion having lower level of fat. Normally oil-in-water type of emulsion having above 15 percent fat. 'Dairy spreads' contain generally butterfat whereas 'non-dairy spreads' contain vegetable fat. These soft spreadable products rich in poly-unsaturated fatty acids (PUFA) are perceived to have better nutritional profile. Evolution of fat spreads has continued along the lines of achieving lower and lower fat levels without losing the age-old sensory appeal of the high-fat products viz., conventional table butter.

History of Fat Spread Development

Emperor Louis Napoleon III of France developed margarine in 1869. During 1886s Hippolyte Mege-Mourie formulated a product, which he named oleomargarine and the fat source, oleo oil derived from beef fat. Margarine quality was improved considerably in 1920s. Hydrogenated vegetable oil were used to greater extend but initially as blend with animal fat, later hydrogenated coconut oil came into wider use. The only major product innovation during this period was addition of vitamins. Margarine must contain an 80 percent fat. Health concern has led to the development of many low fat spread products, which have lower energy content. The mid 1960s saw the introduction of soft margarine made from safflower oil with a high polyunsaturated to saturate fat ratio (P/S) and was an immediate success. These products received considerable publicity in the 1980s with the publication of the COMA (Committee on the Medical Aspects of Food in the UK) report, which promoted the reduction of total fat and saturated fatty acid in the diet.

The attraction for a suitable alternative arises from the fact that spreads can cut both on total fat and saturated fat intake and easy spreadability at refrigerated temperature. The driving force behind development of spreads was the health needs of the human populace. Three phases mark the development of table spreads.

First phase consisted of extended raw material base from original animal body fat to other suitable edible fats such as vegetable oils. Attempt in this direction was greatly facilitated by the process of refining and hydrogenation. This was mainly to increase the availability of other table spreads.

The second phase was related to the compositional aspects fulfilling two needs, one physical and other chemical. With the universal use of house hold refrigerator the butter stored tended to be hard and difficult to spread. To make it softer higher levels of liquid fats/oils were used and special processing conditions have to be applied to attain desired rheological properties.

In the third phase the opportunity afforded by efficient emulsifying agents and process equipments was utilized for making spreads to cover other nutrients such as proteins.

Although milk fat and vegetable fat mixtures, known as "mélanges", have been used over the year, usually with butter fat levels below 10 percent, It was not until mid 1970's that an 80 percent "mélange" and "Bregott" with around 75 percent butter was marketed in Sweden. In the late 1970's the low-protein and high protein "halvarines" were introduced, for the first time in the United Kingdom (UK) with the use of preservatives. By the 1980's the fat levels in most traditional brands started to fall and the ubiquitous reduced 60 percent fat spread' entered the market. The very-low-fat 20 percent fat and 'almost-zero-fat' spreads were introduced in the late 1980's and early 1990's. The first significant cholesterol lowering yellow fat spreads and Benecol was introduced in 2000 by Unilever, UK. Presently, organic spreads have started to appear on the supermarket shelves. The low fat spread market is still at infancy stage in India. Lipton (India) was the first to launch branded margarine (Blue Band) in 1970's. It was a bland white margarine, used mainly for baking with secondary use as bread spread. In Indian market, various brands of table spreads like Amul Lite (Anand milk producers union Ltd.), Blue Band (Lipton), Spread it Margarine (Bharat Margarine Ltd.) and Marigold Margarine (Amrit Banaspati), Chaska Muska and Britannia cheese spread (Britannia) are available which are based on replacement of milk fat to varying degree and having different rheological properties. Considerable efforts have been made in India for development of fat spreads of dairy and non-dairy type using variety of ingredients such as vegetable fat and soy concentrate; cream, vegetable fat and SMP and Cheese, paneer and channa based spread, butter chakka and chhana, cheese and chakka, cheese and butter milk, Ultrafiltration retentate and safflower milk blended with buffalo milk. In the year 2002 the share of dairy spreads in the international yellow fat market was 7 percent by volume while 6 percent by value. During 2005 the value of the margarine and spreads sector increased to some 375 million Euro and this was result of the spreads sector's comparative success, where healthy spreads (such as soya, olive oil and functional spreads) in particular, are forecast to be a real growth area.

Food companies world over have developed numerous substitute products under the name of table spreads which could take care of drawbacks associated with butter in relation to spreadability at low temperature and retention of consistency at ambient temperature. Sophisticated manufacturing techniques have been developed making it possible to have tailor made products.

Table. 5.1: Range of spreadable products

Product	Fat (%)	Saturated fat (g/100g)	Energy (Kcal/100g)
Butter	80.00	54.00	740
Margerine	80.00	16.0-35.0	740
Dairy spread	75.00	28.00	660
Low fat spread	40.00	11.00	400
Very low fat spread	25.00	6.00	275

Compiled from different sources

Definition and Classification

Earlier PFA rules 1954 (as amended in 2006) defined table spread that may contain edible common salt (2%), milk solids not fat, starch (100-150 ppm), diacetyl may be added as flavouring agent (4 ppm) and permitted class II preservatives (1000 ppm) and permitted emulsifier and stabilizers; permitted antioxidants (BHA and TBHQ) not exceeding 0.02 percent of the fat content. It may also contain annatto and/or carotene as colouring agents. It shall be free from animal body fat, mineral oil and wax. Fat should not be more than 80 percent and not less than 40 percent by weight, moisture should not be more than 50 percent and not less than 16 percent by weight. Vegetable fat spread should contain not less than 25 IU synthetic vitamin 'A' per gram. As per Agmark Certification, it should be sold in sealed packages weighing not more than 500 grams.

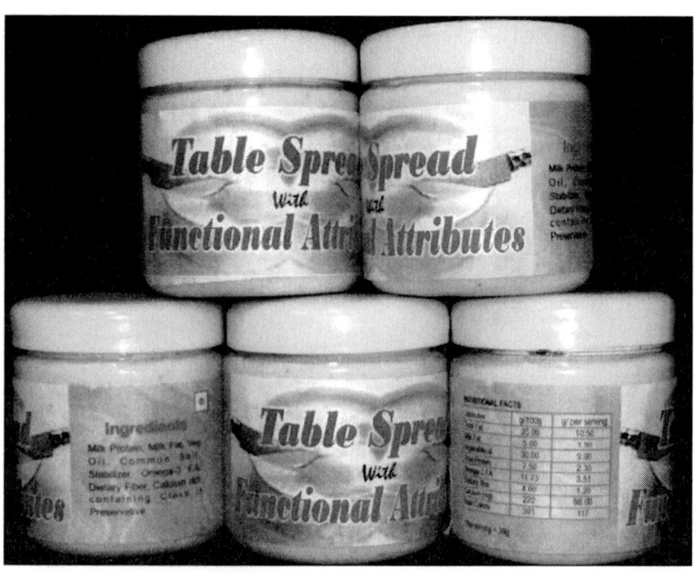

FSSAI Definition for Fat Spread

According to FSSAI, 2011 - Fat spread is a product in the form of water in oil emulsion, Which may contain not more than 80%Fat and not less than 40%Fat by weight, moisture should not be more than 56% and not less than 16% by weight. It may contain edible salt not exceeding 2% by weight in aqueous phase, starch not less than 100ppm and not more than 150ppm, diacetyl may be used as flavouring agent not exceeding 4.0ppm, permitted class II preservatives namely sorbic acid, and its sodium, potassium and calcium salts (calculated as sorbic acid), benzoic acid and its sodium its sodium and potassium salts (calculated as benzoic acid) singly or in combination not exceeding 1000 parts per million by weight. It may contain sequestering agent, permitted emulsifier and stabilizer, permitted antioxidants (BHA or TBHQ) not exceeding 0.02% of the fat content of the spread. It may contain annatto and/or carotene as colouring agents. It shall be free from animal body fat, mineral oil and wax. The vegetable fat spread shall contain not less than 25 IU synthetic vitamin 'A' per gram at the time of packing. Acid value of extracted fat should not be more than 0.5.

Also, FSSAI -2011 prescribes additional specifications based on type of spreads, they are melting point, unsaponifiable matter, acid value and starch content. The melting point of extracted fat shall not be more than 37°C in case of vegetable fat spread (capillary slip method). The unsaponifiable matter of extracted fat shall not be more than 1.5 (for vegetable fat spreads) and 1 percent (for milk fat and mixed fat spreads) by weight. The acid value of extracted fat shall not be more than 0.5. Product shall contain starch not less than 100ppm and not more than 150 ppm. In case of vegetable fat spread it is compulsory to add not less than 25 IU vitamin A.

Margarine: According to FSSAI -2011, there are two types of margarine namely

1. Table margarine and 2. Bakery/Industrial margarine.

Table and industrial margarine are water in oil type emulsions consisting of continuous edible oils and fats and dispersed aqueous phase (water phase). According to FSSAI -2011, it shall be free from rancidity, mineral oil and animal body fats, it shall contain fat not less than 80 percent by weight, moisture not less than 12 percent and not more than 16 percent by weight. It shall contain vitamin-A not less than 30 IU per gram. It may contain common salt not exceeding 2.5 percent. The requirements between table and industrial margarine as per FSSAI -2011 are as follows.

Parameter	Table margarine	Industrial margarine
Addition of colour and flavour	Allowed	Not allowed
Melting point of extracted fat	31°C to 37°C	31°C - 41°C
Unsaponifiable matter of extracted fat	NMT 1.5% by weight	NMT 2.5% by weight if rice bran oil (RBO) is declared on label and NMT 2.0% if RBO is more than 30%
SMP	NMT 2 percent by weight	Not mentioned
Free Fatty Acid	NMT 0.25 per cent oleic acid	NMT 0.25 per cent oleic acid
Acid value	NMT 0.5	NMT 0.5
Starch	NLT 100 ppm and NMT 150 ppm	Not applicable
Package	sold in sealed packages weighingNMT 500gms	Not applicable

Note: NMT: Not more than, NLT: Not less than

Labeling of Fat Spread: The word 'butter' will not be associated while labeling the product. The fat content shall be declared on the label. In mixed fat spread, the milk fat content shall also be declared on the label along with the total fat content.It shall be compulsorily sold in sealed packages weighing not more than 500gram under Agmark certification mark.

Classification of Fat Spreads

FSSAI - 2011 classified fat spreads into three types based on the source of fat.

1. Milk fat spread
2. Mixed fat spread and
3. Vegetable fat spread

Milk fat spreads are made of exclusively milk fat, mixed fat spreads are made of mixture of milk fat with any one or more of hydrogenated, unhydrogenated refined edible vegetable oils or interesterified fat and vegetable fat spreads are made of exclusively vegetable oils and fats (mixture of any two or more of hydrogenated, unhydrogenated refined vegetable oils or interesterfied fat).

Melting point of extracted fat (Capillary slip method) in case of vegetable fat spread should not be more than 37°C.

Table 5.2: Fat content of various spreadable products as per the EU guidelines

Total fat content (percent)	*Type of fat*		
	Pure Milk Fat (100 percent)	Blended fat Non-milk fat	Non-milk fat (MF 0-3 percent)
80-<90	Butter	Blend	Margarine
60-62	Three-quarter fat butter	Three-quarter fat blend	Three-quarter fat margarine
<39-41	Half-fat butter	Half-fat blend	Half-fat margarine
<39	Dairy spread	Blended spread	Fat spread
>41-<60	Dairy spread	Blended spread	Fat spread
>60-<80	Dairy spread	Blended spread	Fat spread

*MF-milk-fat

Source: Fred (2003)

Fat Spread Formulation

Various ingredients for the production of fat spread greatly depend on the type of spread desired i.e. low or high fat, sweetened or salted, spices or flavoured, storage temperature and nutritional aspects etc. Major ingredients commonly used in the preparation of table spreads are milk fat, milk proteins, vegetable fat, emulsifiers, stabilizers, acidulants, salt, colouring agents, flavouring agents, vitamins and antioxidants. The various ingredients are choosen based on type of spread as given in Table 5.3.

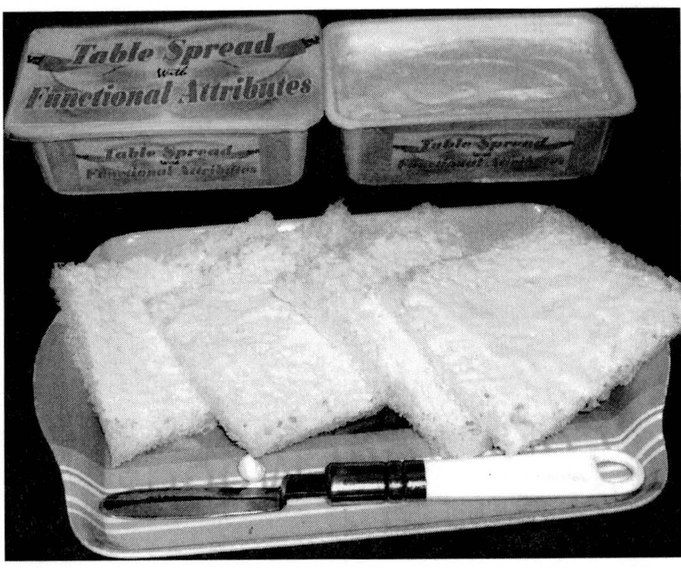

Table 5.3: Typical fat spreads formulations

Spread Type	Fat (%)	Protein (%)	Emulsifier/ emulsifying salt	Stabilizer	Preser- vatives	Colour Flavour and Vitamins
Margarine	>80	0.2	+	-	-	+
Reduced Fat	60-75	0.3	+	-	-	+
Low Fat	38.40	0.2-6.5	+	2"	+	+
Very low Fat	20.25	0-8.3	+	2"	+	+
Oil-in-water type	5.12	12.20	+	2"	2"	+

2"denotes an optional.

Source: (Moran, 1994)

Role and Source of Ingredients

Fat : Fat is a major ingredient of any table spread. The main functions of fat are to provide structure, energy, mouth feel, act as a carrier of flavour and vitamins and as source of essential fatty acids and fat-soluble vitamins. It is the major ingredient contributing to the viscosity and body of the spread. It governs consistency, spreadability, creaminess, firmness, plasticity depending on amount of fat and type of fat. The rigidity of emulsion depends on the size of the oil droplets and partly on how tightly they are packed. The major criterion for oil selection for spreads and margarine is the degree of unsaturation in the constituent fatty acids. Source of fat includes - cream, butter, butter oil and vegetable fat/oils. When vegetable oils are used it could be as such or after modification including butter fat.

Milk fat : Cream as a source of fat with a fat content of 40-50% is generally used in fat spreads. However, high fat cream containing 50-75% fat can also be used. Spread with 20 percent fat cream show sour curdy taste while, 30 percent fat cream had optimum smoothness and resistance for spreading. Butter as a source of fat is used in preparation of reduced fat or low-fat spreads and have been observed to provide firmer body as compared to cream based spreads. The low-fat butter spread is an emulsion of fat with an aqueous phase of non-fat ingredients. Butter worked under vacuum and blended with caseinates as aqueous phase with homogenization has also been used for manufacture of table spreads. Depending on availability, butter-oil too has been used extensively as a source of milk fat in the manufacture of low fat table spreads.

Milk fat-vegetable oil blends : The demand for low calorie product containing high poly-unsaturated fatty acids has given birth to blended spreads. For this purpose various vegetable oils like sunflower, corn, soybean and groundnut oils are preferred. Milk fat fractions / vegetable oil fractions can also be used. To improve the spreadability of the product at refrigerated temperature, butterfat has been blended with vegetable oil. This also helped to raise the level of polyunsaturated fat in the product. Cream/butter have been blended with single or different vegetable oils in desired proportions for the production of blended fat spreads. Table spreads containing 20-70% fat were manufactured using blends comprising of 10-90% milk fat and 90-10% non milk fat. An artificial butter flavoured spreads have been made using 50:50 blend of hydrogenated vegetable fat and soy oil. Good quality low fat spread can be prepared from safflower oil and buffalo fat blend (50:50) with addition of 1.5 percent common salt, 1.0 percent emulsifier (tri-sodium citrate) and 10 percent ripened cheese and pH adjusted to 5.5. This resulted in a product with significant increase in scores of various sensory attributes.

Modified milk fat : Production of spread by altering fatty acid composition or other beneficial milk fat components would be an ideal nutritional spread for consumer. Fractionated fats using low melting fat fractions have been employed in manufacture of dairy spreads to produce specific desirable characteristics. Fractionation is apparently the best alternative for improving functional properties of butter. Recombined butter using fractionated fat have been developed that exhibits good spreadability at 4°C and maintained its physical structure at room temperature. Cold spreadable butter spread without any adverse effect on the flavour has been made by blending butter fat with structured lipid (80:20) was synthesized from canola oil with sn-1, 3 specific lipase form *Rhizomucor miehei*.

Monounsaturated fatty acids (MUFA) spread : Oils rich in monounsaturated fatty acids e.g. peanut, canola, rice bran, high-oleic safflower and sesame oils with their oleic content in the range of 41.2-79.7 percent and saturated fatty acid 16 percent or less have become particularly desirable in fat blends for low-fat spreads.

Trans-fatty acid (TFA)-free spread : The negative health image of TFA among the consumers of fat spreads has led to development of several low or no *tarns* fat blends. The oil processing technologies which can yield fats with, the desired physical properties without producing TFA have been sought to improve the health value of spreads. Interesterification is one of the tool to reduce the TFA in oils and fats. Non-dairy spreads low in TFA can be obtained by using tropical oils such as palm oil, palm kernel oil and coconut oil. Interesterified mixture of coconut oil, palm oil and palm stearin (the last obtained as a solid fat upon fractionation of palm oil) has been used in preparation of soft margarines. Spreads prepared from blend containing liquid oil, 3-10 percent a fully hydrogenated palmitic fat and less than 3 percent *trans*-fatty acids have been developed. Similarly zero-TFA spreads have also been produced employing interesterification approach.

Fat replacers : Development and use of vide varieties of food ingredients called fat replacers have made it possible the production of many low fat or zero fat spreads. There are two primary types of fat replacer i.e. energy free fat substitutes and energy reduced fat mimetics. The fat substitutes are neither digested nor absorbed and therefore contribute no fat, energy and cholesterol in the diet. Such fat substitutes includes carbohydrate fatty acids polyesters, malonate esters, esterified propoxylated glycerol etc. Fat memetics have the ability to replace mouth feel of fats. These are protein based, carbohydrate or starch or cellulose based. Some of the protein based fat replacers are – Simlesse, Trailblazer and Finnesse. They are bland in taste and soluble in water. They provide spreadability and appearance to the low fat spreads. Cellulose based fat replacers contribute only to creamy mouth feel to the product.

Protein : Proteins modulates organoleptic, functional and nutritional properties of spreads. This non fatty constituent of spread plays an important role in texture of spreads. Protein helps in emulsifying fat and adsorption of water thereby providing physical stability to the final product. The type and level of protein affects body and texture of low fat spreads. Apart from contributing flavour, it acts as preservative by sequestering metals that promote oxidation. Milk Protein in the form of skim milk, concentrated skim milk, skim milk powder (SMP), whey powder, whey protein concentrate (WPC), casienates, co-precipitate, butter milk, butter milk powder, whey powder, and ultra-filterate milk protein concentrate may be used for manufacture of table spreads. Milk protein, from different sources, and at different levels ranging from 5-15% have been used for manufacture of different spreads. However, 6% level has been found to provide good binding effect, spreadability and stability with better body and texture characteristics. SMP is frequently used as non fat solids source in low-fat spread. Addition of 5 percent to 10 percent SMP enhanced flavour and texture characteristics of the spread where as 15 percent had an adverse effect on mouth feels. Use of whey protein concentrate prepared by UF process had the ability to improve the body of the product with the least wheying off. Replacement of non-fat milk solids with dried whey protein concentrate has more potential not only to improve the quality of the product, but also to reduce the cost of the product. Whey protein concentrate containing 75 percent of protein exhibited desirable functional properties such as excellent water holding capacity, solubility, emulsification, elasticity, viscosity and organoleptic characteristics. Incorporation of concentrated buttermilk as a protein source in the spread results in stable emulsion. The emulsion stability of low fat, water-in- oil spread using buttermilk powder was found to be superior to that of spread from SMP. Acceptable quality table spread can be manufactured by using buttermilk solids at 20 percent in final product. Milk protein can be replaced with vegetable proteins like, soy protein isolate, which have been found to improve organoleptic, functional and nutritional properties of blended spreads.

Emulsifiers : These are important additives that hold the emulsion ingredients together and avoid destabilization. Emulsifiers are essential to maintain fat in continuous structure, especially during manufacture. They contribute towards initial nucleation of high melting tri-glyceride crystals during crystallization process. Such crystals can preserve the emulsion structure by forming solid shells around the aqueous phase droplets and are the main stabilizing system in the product. Fat soluble emulsifiers are preferred because of fat is the major portion in the product also fat present in continuous phase. Monoglycerides of saturated fatty acids, unsaturated fatty acids, lecithin, egg yolk solids are used at a level of 0.1 to 0.6%. These emulsifiers help in reducing the size of aqueous droplets and create stabilizing films at the water/oil interface, so that product will be softer and spreadable. The type and level of emulsifier is govern by the type of emulsion (whether oil-in-water or oil-in-water type), nature of ingredients and processing conditions. Recently, consumer tests have shown a certain degree of concern on the issue of additive free dairy foods. In spreads the use of emulsifiers can be eliminated at least in part by using residual levels of such emulsifiers present in natural fats. Dairy cream when used as an ingredient may provide sufficient amount of natural emulsifier to stabilize the system. Usage of ultra-filtrate retentate as a source of protein, acts as an emulsifier. Thus such products do not require any stabilizers and emulsifiers and are free from these additives. Using membrane separation processes the components of milk such as butter serum, whey, ultrafiltered skim milk protein, whey proteins, casiens and fat globule membrane proteins can be obtained which are having good emulsifying properties.

Stabilizers : These are basically hydrocolloids and have a tendency to hold water. Hydrocolloids are mostly complex carbohydrates, which are used to improve consistency, textural characteristics (rheological properties) and overall appearance without changing nutritional values and sensory qualities of food products. They can be added in various combinations and phases of production and may have different final effects. Generally, they are added at the rate of 0.1-0.5 percent. Their usage in spread preparation may result in increased firmness of the product. As the fat spreads contain 30-50%moisture, excessive free moisture may lead to poor consistency and plasticity defects in the product. Stabilizers having high water holding capacities contribute towards improving the textural characteristics of spreads. Especially important in reduced/low fat spreads wherein high water holding ability of stabilizer improves body & texture of the spread. They help in increasing the viscosity and also to inhibit the coalescence of aqueous phase droplets during processing. Carboxy methy cellulose(CMC), modified starch, modium alginate, starch, vegetable gums like locust bean gum and guar gum, carragennan, gelatin can be used as stabilizers at a level of 0.1 to 0.5%. They provide fine, uniform texture and excellent moisture retention properties. Gelatin and CMC individually or in combination have been most extensively used in spreads resulting in pleasant taste, good consistency and spreadability at a wide temperature range and least wheying off. Higher concentration of gelatin however, may result in crumbly body of the spread.

Acidifying agents : Owing to their high moisture content, spreads in general have low storage stability. Creating a low pH in the system may help extent the shelf life of the product by retarding bacterial growth. For this reason certain acidogenic substances are added such as lactic, acetic, citric and salts of glucono-delta-lactones (GDL) are used to control the pH of the system. Thus the roles of acidifying agents, added to table spread, are acidification, flavour enhancement and microbial inhibition. An important property of organic acid is their effectiveness as antimicrobial agents. Indeed, this is true for all organic acid used in the formulation of edible table spread. Acidification of spread with lactic acid resulted in improvement in body and tended to impart slightly tart flavour to a low-fat spread product. The reaction of the spread mix is often the deciding factor as to what type of emulsion would be obtained. For best body and least weeping a pH of 5.7-5.9 is kept of the system. Lower pH would result in synersis while high pH would result in formation of oil-in-water (O/W) type emulsion.

Sodium chloride (common salt) – Addition of common salt generally improves flavour acceptability of spreads. In addition it helps to inhibit the growth of bacteria and fungi and thereby acts as a preservative. The usual range of salt addition varies from 0.5%-1.25%. Good shelf life can be obtained by using 0.5% level of salt. Higher salt level does not have any perceptible influence on body and texture (firmness and stickness) of the product. It slightly improves flavour, spreadability and colour of resultant spread. It also plays a significant role in increasing the viscosity of the spreads containing casienates as protein source. Higher salt concentration result in swelling and partial unfolding of casein aggregates thereby increasing voluminosity of protein and hence the viscosity of the system.

Flavourings : During the production of table spreads variety of raw materials are blended to give the final product of required properties. The acceptability of newly developed product largely depends on the pleasant flavour together with rheological properties that are suited to consumers need. A variety of natural, nature identical and artificial flavouring compounds have been used in table spreads. To mimic butter like flavour starter distillates, cultured butter milk and ripened cream have been used. These compounds have been used in the range of 1-1.5%. Amongst artificial flavouring compounds diacetyl (15ppm), butterbuds (1.5%) and butardol (0.23%) have been used to simulate butter like flavour. For spreads having cheese like flavour cheese flavour concentrates may be used or it can be achieved by adding cheese directly into the spread mix. Commercial cheese flavour concentrates in powdered form may be employed in low fat spreads. For direct addition of cheese satisfactory flavour can be obtained by adding well ripened Cheddar, smoked Cheddar or blue cheese at the rate of 20% of the finished product. Due to consumers inclination towards natural flavouring compounds, usage of spices and seasonings such as cummins, black pepper, garlic and ginger may also be used for flavouring of spreads. The mixture of cumin and black pepper in the ratio of 2:1 is quite acceptable and compatible with the spread.

Colourants : Colour marks the impression on the consumers, without proper colouring, the product appears lifeless and unattractive. Two types of colour, namely annatto and β-carotene are added. Other approved colour for used in the edible table spreads are turmeric, β-apo-8' Carotenal and its esters (CAC, 2004). A salient feature of β-carotene as a colourant, is that besides being nutritionally important, it enhances the oxidative stability of the fat products. Annatto colour is used in low fat spreads at the rate of less than 0.01 to 0.3

percent. Among several oil-soluble and water-soluble colourants, a mixture of oil soluble butter annatto (0.15 percent) and β-carotene (10 mg/kg) imparted an acceptable yellow shade in an o/w spread.

Preservatives: Due to high moisture content table spreads generally have short shelf life. Table spreads in general undergo microbial spoilage although oxidative deteriorations have also been reported. At ambient temperature spreads do not have appreciable stability. It is for these reasons addition of some kind of preservative becomes necessary. In addition to heat treatment, various preservative are also added to spreads which includes sorbic acid, benzoic acid and their salts of sodium, potassium and calcium; nisin and propionate etc. The antimicrobial system possessed by lactic acid bacteria offers scope for the development of an effective natural preservative process for application in foods.

Sorbic acid, an antimycotic agent, is a permitted food preservative and is most effective fat-soluble preservative. It has been used in the range of 0.03-0.1 percent in various spread formulations. At 0.1% level sorbic acid suppresses microbial growth and retard oxidation. Inhibition of yeast and mould growth may be achieved by addition of potassium sorbate. Keeping quality of spread increase with addition of potassium sorbate. It acted not only as mould inhibitor but also acted as flavour releasing agent. Benzoic acid imparts maximum antimicrobial activity in the pH range 2.5 to 4 and is most effective against yeast and bacteria. The recommended level of sodium benzoate is 0.1 percent Bacterial and mould induced spoilage may be retarded by addition of sodium benzoate and sodium propionate in the ratio of 2:1. A preservative mixture of sorbic acid, benzoic acid and potassium sorbate at the rate of 0.05% each exhibit greater protective effect when used at 0.1% level. However, FSSAI -2011 permitted to add benzoic acid and sorbic acid and its salts of sodium, potassium and calcium as preservatives in fat spread with maximum concentration of 1000 ppm in terms of sodium benzoate.

In recent years consumers have been demanding a reduction in the use of chemicals preservative in their foods because of potential health risks. In response, manufacturers have been looking for alternative technologies that will preserve the freshness, flavour, texture and nutrient value of their product. The biopreservative viz: Bacteriocin, Nisin, Microgard, Reuterin and Pimaricin, etc. added to various dairy products has yielded highly promising results and enhanced shelf life of product. The biopreservative MicroGardä has a wide antimicrobial spectrum including some gram-negative bacteria, yeast and fungi. MicroGardä is approved by Food Drug Administration, USA. It is added to a variety of dairy products such as cottage cheese and yoghurt at a concentration of 1.0 percent. It inhibits viable yeasts and protects from spoilage by gram negative psychrotrophic bacreria which grow out following pH increase as a result of yeast growth. It has been suggested by the manufacturer that MicroGardä is typically added to the fat spread at the rate of 0.5 to 1 percent. Another biopreservative of promise is the Nisin that has been used since long in dairy foods. Addition of 1465 ppm of nisin, accepted for food use, resulted in the spread showing no sign of bacterial spoilage after 6 weeks at 4.4°C.

Method of Manufacture of Spreads

Given below are the steps that may be followed during preparation of table spreads

1. ***Preparation of fat phase*** : Fat phase is prepared using suitable oil blends, hydrogenated or partially hydrogenated refined oils. Usually it is prepared in double jacketed vat which have stirring heating facility. Temperature of the oil blend is then increased to 60°C. Minor ingredients such as emulsifier like lecithin, oil soluble flavour and colour are then dissolved in the fat phase. An oil-soluble flavour (butter flavour) and colour (annatto or β-carotene) are added to achieve product which taste and look like butter. Antioxidants like vitamin E (tocopherol), butylated hydroxyl anisole (BHA) and tertiary butyl hydroquinone (TBHQ) are also oil soluble. In addition, β-carotene has pro-vitamin A activity.

2. ***Preparation of aqueous phase*** : It is prepared by taking calculated quantity of water in multipurpose vat and then rise the temperature of water to 40°C. Then water soluble ingredients like preservative, salt, whey powder, skimmed milk powder or other types of milk can be added. Stabiliser(s) are needed in order to have the necessary stability in the final crystallised product and also to hold the water. Water-soluble flavour and colour can also be added, but are primarily used in low fat spreads. Alginates, pectin and carrageenans have a good water binding effect and gives stable emulsions.

3. ***Heat treatment (Pasteurization)*** : Both fat as well aqueous phases are heat treated separately, to ensure safety of the product and to minimize microbial contamination. The time temperature combinations used are 75°C for 30 minutes, 85°C for 5 minutes and 95°C for no hold followed

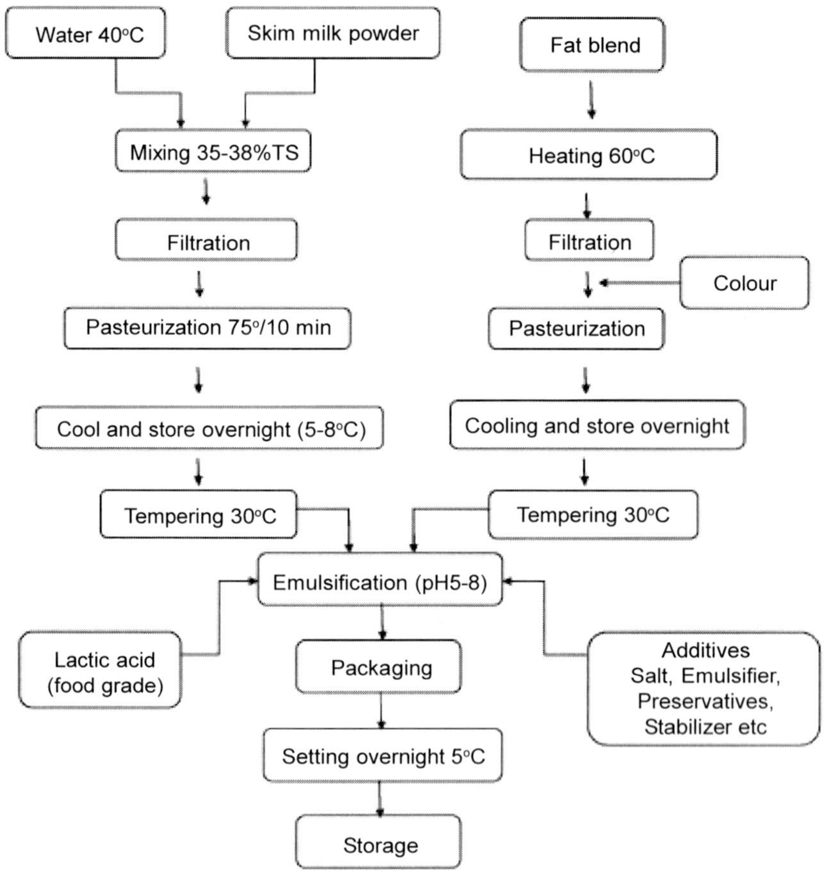

Fig. 5.1: Flow diagram for manufacture of table spread

by prompt cooling of aqueous phase to less than 40°C or 4°C (in case if blending is scheduled later) and fat phase to around 40°C (temperature should be sufficient to keep fat phase in liquid state before blending).

4. ***Emulsion preparation*** : This is a blending process wherein water phase is mixed into oil phase with high speed stirrer using high shear mixer to form an emulsion. After mixing temperature of the blend is maintained at 40°C-50°C, then it is pumped to cooling unit.

5. ***Cooling*** : Cooling is carried out in tubular heat exchanger with continuous scraper blade rotating at rpm of 300-800 continuously to increase the heat transfer rate. Ammonia or Freon is used as refrigerant at about -10°C to -20°C. This induces crystallization of fat and nuclei formation. Coolant temperature, shaft speed, product flow rate acts as controls in this process for desired product consistency and texture.

6. ***Working*** : Working helps in prevents the growth of fat crystals further and also slight raise in temperature during working helps in formation of desired fat crystal structure, it was reported that alpha polymorph crystals are rearranged to beta prime crystal polymorph during working.
7. ***Resting*** : After proper working the prepared spread is allowed to rest for some time. This resting is carried out to develop the desired firmness before packaging.
8. ***Packaging*** : Moisture and air proof containers are required to pack this fat rich product. Suitable packaging materials for this purpose are polystyrene based/polypropylene based cups or tubs, polyethylene coated paper packs along with parchment paper. Air tight food grade PET jars of 200g capacity is the preferred packaging material for table spreads. For larger packing of 400g polystyrene based/polypropylene based cups are also used. Stick type margarine is packed similar to butter – parchment paper is used as primary packaging material and supported by outer polyethylene coated paper board.

Recent Trends in Spreads and Margarine Development

Attempts to improve the nutritional status of edible table spreads have focused on reducing total fat and cholesterol contents, changing the fatty acid profile and eliminating trans-fatty acids. The positive impact of some of these compositional changes on consumer health has resulted in the use of spreads

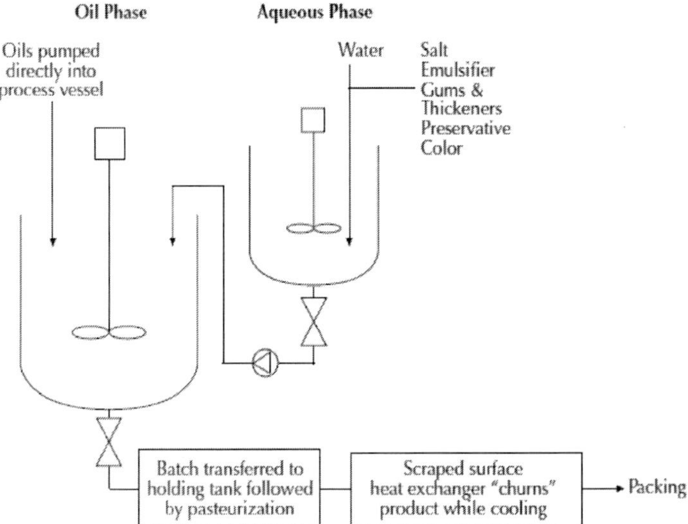

Fig. 5.2: Schematic diagram for manufacture of fat spread

with functional ingredients that could prevent the ever-increasing coronary heart disease (CHD) problems. The demand for such products is likely to escalate in the near future. It is time for the dairy industry to plunge into low fat spreads with functional attributes for health conscious customers and encourage the use of dairy by-products and functional nutrients as ingredients in composite food products. Research potential exists in the field of table spread manufacture with improved characteristics through incorporation of various functional ingredients. Addition of functional ingredients viz. omega-3 fatty acid, dietary fiber, pre- and probiotic, plant sterol, vitamins and essential minerals can be exploited for their health benefits.

Low fat spreads : The term 'low-fat dairy spread' are the products, which contain only dairy ingredients, and have less fat than butter and margarine. Low-fat spreads of both dairy and non-dairy types have been known since late sixties. Dairy spreads containing 39-41 percent fat are sometimes termed as 'half-fat butter' while those in which caloric reduction is at least 33 percent are termed as 'reduced calorie spreads'. Accordingly, a range of spreadable fat products varying widely in their fat content are identified under the EU guidelines (Table 6.1). In general terminology, products with 40 percent or less are known as 'low fat spread', product containing 5-15 percent fat or even less fat as 'very low fat spreads' and the spreads with extremely low fat content are sometimes called 'ultra-low-fat spreads'.

Fortified fat spreads & margarine: Foods fortified with one or more nutrients with functional properties could play an important role in meeting the demands for optimal health. None of the table spreads which are available in Indian market has functional features. Addition of functional ingredients viz. omega-3 fatty acid, dietary fiber, pre and probiotic, plant sterol, vitamins and minerals essential can be exploited for their health benefits. Spreads and margarine are good vehicles for fortification of fat soluble vital components.

i. ***Fortification with Omega-3 Fatty Acids*** : A reduced- fat margarine based on rapeseed oil with a low saturated fat level, high monounsaturated fat level, and omega-3 fatty acids was commercially introduced in Denmark in 1995. It contained a small amount of un-hydrogenated fish oil (giving 0.2 g long-chain omega-3 fatty acids per 15 g of the spread) and the spread was claimed to be stable and free from fishy flavour. A low fat spread containing un-hydrogenated fish oil that is free from trans fatty acids and enriched with long chain omega-3 fatty acids from fish oil have been reported. To achieve a more desirable ratio of dietary omega-3 to omega-6 PUFAs, consumption of fish and omega-3-rich seed oils, such as canola, soy and flaxseed and spreads made with these oils have been encouraged. This would help to increase the á-linolenic acid from about 500 mg to 1,600 mg per day and is expected to result in reduced risk for heart attacks. A daily Consumption of 30 g portion of omega-3 containing fat spread would provide 0.25 g of EPA and DHA, significantly increasing long-chain omega-3 levels in the average diet. A buttery spread containing omega-3 fatty acid and fortified with 15% or more of vitamin D, E, B_6 and B_{12} have been shown to help lower the risk for heart disease and boost immune system.

ii. ***Fortification with dietary fiber*** : Both inulin and oligofructose have been demonstrated to be effective prebiotic. Because of their recognized prebiotic properties, principally the selective stimulation of colonic bifidobacteria, therefore, both are being increasingly used in new food product developments. Food manufacturers usually decide to use inulin properties for their nutritional or the technological reasons. The unique properties of inulin have resulted in introduction of rapidly growing number of inulin containing table spreads, butter-like products and dairy spreads. The use of inulin in a low fat spread formulation, as a structuring agent, is said to improve spreadability, provide creamy, fat-like mouthfeel, better flavour release and processing stability. Excellent results may be obtained in water-in-oil spreads with a fat content ranging from 20 to 60 percent, as well as in water-continuous formulations containing 15 percent fat or less. Inulin containing spread (Actiline) manufactured by Belgium Company Vamdermoortele is available in European market. Inulin at 4-5 percent gave better body-texture and spreadability than oat fiber. Inulin intake up to 20 g/day has been found to decrease plasma triglycerides and cholesterol. It is also expected to improvise glucose tolerance in diabetics.

iii. ***Fortification with vitamins and minerals*** : The low fat spread has been used as vehicles for folic acid fortification. The absorption of folic acid from low-fat spread, fortified with 200 µg folic acid, although lower than from a tablet, is effective. These results suggest that low-fat spreads, typically associated with fat-soluble vitamins (A, D, E) fortification, may also be considered feasible as vehicles for folic acid fortification. A number of calcium-supplemented foods, including spreads, came on the market. A spread enriched in vitamin D and calcium is available Netherland market. The manufacturer claims to supply 15 percent of recommended dietary allowances (RDA) calcium intake from 25 g spread daily. Low fat spreads might thus be viewed positively as vehicle for lipolytic nutrients without excessive lipid and can contribute to fulfillment of the recommended daily intake of A, D and E vitamins. A highly nutrient-dense (HND) spread obtained by blending skim milk powder with peanut butter and powdered lactoserum and containing 10 percent protein and 57 percent fat in addition to mineral and vitamins, used to deliver multiple micronutrients in concentrated forms, was found to serve as highly effective supplement to the local diet. An amount of HND spread need to deliver a daily dose of micronutrients can vary from 10 g to 100 g per day. A new approach is to develop a fortified food with lower nutrient density. Supplementation with zinc and possibly iron and vitamin B_{12} was shown to improve linear growth of children in deficient populations. For most vitamins and minerals, fortification amounts were 1.5–3 times the dietary reference intakes.

iv. ***Fortification with antioxidant*** : Spreads are good vehicle for carrying of fat-soluble antioxidants, because antioxidants are needed for efficient absorption. Antioxidants are substances that, when present at much lower concentrations than an oxidizable substrate, significantly delay or prevent its oxidation. Certain essential antioxidants like vitamin E, beta- carotene and vitamin C, protect cells from damage by oxidants.

(a) ***Vitamin E*** : The principal source of vitamin E is vegetable oils. Table spreads made from vegetable oils are therefore good dietary sources of vitamin E. Spreads containing 0.6 g of vitamin E per gram of linoleic acid could contribute towards lowering a risk of CHD. The effect of moderate doses of a combination of vitamin E and carotenoids, incorporated into a food product, on lipid peroxidation in healthy persons showed that consuming 25 g/day of spread containing 43 mg α-tocopherol and 0.45 mg carotenoids resulted in an increase in plasma α-tocopherol concentrations from 31 to 32 mmol/L, with significant increases in concentrations of α-carotene and lutein. Furthermore, consumption of spread containing 111 mg α-tocopherol and 1.24 mg carotenoids significantly reduced concentrations of the plasma lipid peroxidation.

(b) ***Carotenoids*** : The major dietary carotenoids are α-and β-carotene, β-cryptoxanthin, lycopene, lutein and zeaxanthin Lycopene may have more promise than b-carotene. Intake of lycopene is largely from tomatoes. It has potent antioxidant properties, particularly in quenching singlet oxygen. Beta-carotene and lycopene are fat-soluble compounds and may be applied in spreads. However, they impart orange or red colour in spreads, which limits their application. This could be overcome by encapsulation of b-carotene and lycopene, into liposomes which may reduce colouring. The major dietary carotenoids like a and b carotene, lycopene and zeaxanthin have been used for enrichment of fat spreads and used for treatment of vitamin A deficiency.

v. ***Fortification with plant sterol/stanols*** : During 1980s, the cholesterol lowering effects of foods fortified with plant sterols (Ps) were well recognized. Margarines and butter appear as ideal vehicles for incorporating plant sterols because of their strong lypophilic nature. There are now available margarines that have no trans fatty acids. Some also have added stanol esters, which are products of vegetable oils that can actually lower serum cholesterol. Such product is sold under the trade names Benecol, Smart Balance Plus, and Take Control. Benecol, a margarine containing plant stanol ester launched in 1995 by Raisio group, Finland, is an example of a functional food that has been shown to effectively lower serum total and low-density lipoprotein (LDL) cholesterol levels. Fat spreads containing 11 percent phytosterol from soybean and was partly esterified with sunflower oil, with a cholesterol-lowering claim has been developed. A similar preparation 'Monihyva' containing plant sterol was launched in Finnish market and claim to lower LDL cholesterol. In Europe, the average consumption of butter or margarine is about 25 g/person/day and, according to the previous opinion of the Committee on the safety for the use of phytosterol esters in yellow fat spreads, the sterol-enriched margarines may contain up to 2 g of plant sterols or stanols per daily portion. Recommended spread intake of 15 g/day enriched with phytosterol was effective in lowering plasma total cholesterol (TC) and LDL cholesterol (LDL-C) concentrations by 5.8 and 9.1 percent. Consumption of a phytosterol enriched spread effectively lowered plasma TC, LDL-C, Plasma apolipoprotein B (apo B) and remnant-like particle cholesterol (RLP-C) regardless of baseline plasma .total cholostrol. A 35 percent fat spread enriched with 8.3 percent of plant sterols, when consumed 25 g/day resulted in daily intake of about 2g plant sterol and found to be effective in lowering blood levels of total and LDL cholesterol and apolioprotein B, thereby reducing the risk of heart disease. Spreads containing 8 g plant sterol (or stanol) per 100 g have been developed. Consumption of 25 g of such a spread would ensure the recommended daily intake of 2-3g of plant sterols, with an expected lowering of total cholesterol by about 10 percent and LDL cholesterol by 10-15 percent, with a minimal change in HDL cholesterol. When plant sterols/stanols are added to foods such as margarine/ spread with an average dose of 2.4 g/day, lowering was 9.9 percent for LDL-C.

vi. ***Fortification with probiotic and other*** : A reduced fat dairy spread has been developed with added viable, mixed-strain and potentially probiotic culture. The spread contained a lipid phase of anhydrous milk fat, a hard milk fat fraction and soybean oil (66:26:8) combined with emulsifier at 0.4 percent (w/w), and of aqueous phase. Probiotic bacteria added were *Lactobacillus casei* ACA-DC 212.3 and *Bifidobacterium infantis* ATCC 25962. Using process involving pre-emulsification pasteurisation, emulsification, processing and packaging under nitrogen atmosphere, and use of a hydrocolloid-stabilized aqueous phase to achieve acceptable strain viability (with a viable count of 10^5 cfu/ml). A spread (low calorie margarine), in which the fat phase comprised essentially monoglycerides, was reported to be useful as nutritional supplement for consumers with digestive disorders. Similarly medium-chain triacylglycerols based on caprylic and capric acids, which are rapidly absorbed, have been incorporated into margarines meant for patients with impaired fat metabolism.

Types of Spread Based on Source of Fat

Cream spread – Process has been standardized for the manufacture of low calorie butter spread from cream containing 50 percent less fat than in conventional butter. It has been purposed that good quality low fat spread can be prepared from safflower oil and buffalo fat blend (50:50) with addition of 1.5 percent common salt, 1.0 percent emulsifier (trisodium citrate) and 10 percent ripened cheese and pH adjusted to 5.5. This resulted in a product with significant increase in scores of various sensory attributes. Cream spread prepared with 30 percent fat cream was found to have optimum smoothness and resistance for spreading.

Butter spreads : Butter has often been used as a base for low-fat spreads by many investigators. The low-fat butter spread is an emulsion of fat with an aqueous phase of non-fat ingredients. Butter worked under vacuum and blended with caseinates as aqueous phase with homogenization may produce good textural characteristics in spread. Ingredients like cream, stabilizers, emulsifier, flavour, colour blended at an elevated temperature and passed through high pressure Tubular chiller and Pin Rotor machine have been used as a method of spread preparation.

Vegetable oil and milk fat blend spread : To improve the spreadability of the product at refrigerated temperature, butterfat has been blended with vegetable oil. This also helped to raise the level of polyunsaturated fat in the product. On the basis of flavour and fatty acid composition, corn, safflower, soybean, mustard and groundnut oils have been preferred for spreads. Soybean oil is most preferred for the preparation of spreads, as its application improves the stability and flavour and makes the emulsion stronger as compared to cottonseed oil. The effect of using mixed fat blend (milk fat – canola oil) on physical property of spread shows that hardness index of spread decreased with increase in the proportion of oil in the blend. Replacement of 30 percent of milk fat with sunflower oil and found to improve the spreadability of resultant spread at low temperature. A mixture containing 20-50 percent of vegetable oil and 0-50 percent butter oil has been used for the production of plastic spread. A Table spread with good body and texture could be prepared using a fat blend containing 70 percent groundnut oil and 30percent milk fat. Mixed fat spread containing 10 percent milk fat and 49 percent vegetable oil (Amul light) was launched by Gujarat Cooperative Milk Federation.

Manufacturing Process of Blended Fat Spread

For preparation of blended spreads following steps are involved

1. Selection of suitable source/s of protein and fat from different sources consisting of 1-3 components.
2. Taking calculated amount of protein source and blending with fat source by way of slow addition, in a suitable food blender, to form an oil-in-water type emulsion.
3. Adding calculated amount of stabilizer (0.3-.05%) and salt (1%) and mix until proper dispersion is obtained.
4. Pre-heating the emulsion at 60-65°C and homogenizing at 250-300 + 50 bar in two stage homogenizer.

5. Adding flavour of choice and blend to uniformely distribute throughout the emulsion.
6. Pasteurizing the dispersion at 85ºC for 15-20 minutes and allow to cool at room temperature.
7. Hot fill the resultant spread and store at 8-10ºC.

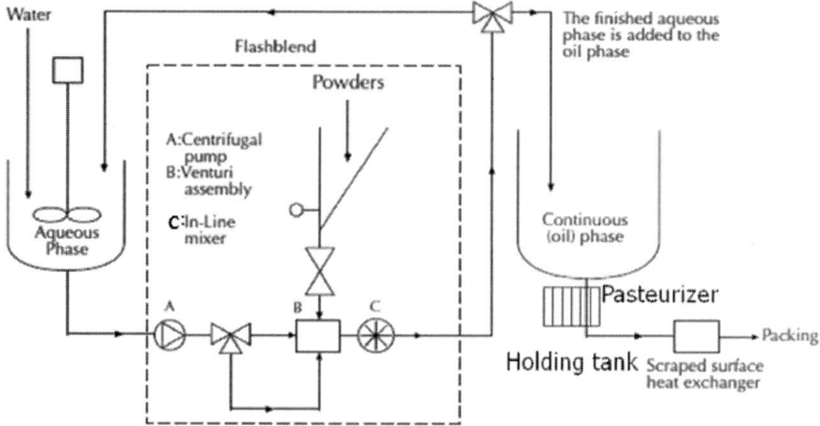

Fig. 5.3: Schematics for venturi assembly system

Packaging

Moisture and air proof containers are required to pack this fat rich product. Suitable packaging materials for this purpose are polystyrene based/ polypropylene based cups or tubs, polyethylene coated paper packs along with parchment paper. Air tight food grade PET jars of 200 g capacity is the preferred packaging material for table spreads. For larger packing of 400 g polystyrene based/polypropylene based cups are also used.

Shelf life and Storage

Storage stability of the spread depends on the type of treatment applied to the product. At ambient temperature spreadable products do not have any appreciable shelf stability. Basically table spreads undergo chemical and microbiological spoilage. Microorganisms that cause spoilage in butter have been implicated with spoilage of table spread. It is well known that lower the temperature of storage the longer is the self life for most of the food product. Depending upon the temperature of storage, the shelf life of table spreads may vary from 10-12 days at ambient temperature and 30-90 days at refrigerated temperature. Refrigerated Storage is preferred for longer shelf life. The shelf life may varies from 90 days to 180 days when stored at 5^0C. Processing conditions & formulations also have influence on the shelf life of the product.

Changes During Storage

Basically table spreads undergo chemical and microbiological spoilage. Microorganisms that cause spoilage in butter have been implicated with spoilage of table spread. However vegetable oils are typically more resistant to lipolytic break down than milk fat. Spreads generally have a shelf life of 10-12 days at 30°C; 28-30 days at 20°C and 60-90 days at 4-6°C.

Chemical Changes

Moisture and water activity of any product is one of the most important factors affecting the shelf life. The increase in moisture content from 12 to 35 percent changed all the rheological characteristics of butter. However, spreads having usually low moisture content (25%) have also sometimes show poor shelf life. A minimum water activity (a_w) is required at which certain types of microorganism can grow. In general bacteria require the higher a_w and moulds can grow at lower a_w. Lower a_w restricts the type of microorganism capable of growth. The increase in the pH was attributed to production of acid by concomitant increase in total viable count as well as yeast and mould count. An increase in the pH value of low calorie butter spreads during storage was reported. However, no relationship between pH and storage period could be established. Titartable acidity greatly influences the flavour score of the dairy spreads. The change in titratable acidity is the result of various biochemical changes caused due to the microbial action. The titartable acidity may remain unchanged for a period of 10 - 12 weeks and then afterwards it increases progressively. Increase in FFA and peroxide value could be due to fat degradation caused, presumably, by microorganism. However this increase could effectively be controlled by using preservatives. The oxidative deterioration of Poly unsaturated Fatty Acid in the spread is generally revealed by increase in TBA value during storage. Fat content in butter spreads ranging for 35-40 percent could give a satisfactory stable emulsion while lower fat levels resulted in either exudation of moisture or unstable emulsions. Spreads may exhibit wheying off during storage depending on the stabilizer and period / temperature of storage. Use of monoglyceride and citrate in soy-based spreads retards the viscosity at the processing temperature and oiling off in the finished product. Penetration value, extrusion thrust and extruder fraction are often used for studying the rheological characteristics of the spreads. Blending butter and cream (with 40% fat) in equal proportion would give optimal rheological properties. Incorporation of safflower or sunflower oil in buffalo cream in the preparation of dairy spread may result in soft body as revealed by increase in the penetration value and decrease in extruder thrust and extruder friction.

Microbiological Changes

The microflora of edible table spreads reflects the quality of the ingredients, the sanitary conditions of the equipment used in the manufacturer and the environmental and sanitary conditions during packaging, storage and handling. Pasteurization of the aqueous phase prior to emulsification and of the emulsion during processing causes a significant reduction in the number of most heat resistant microorganism. The SPC of the spread ranged from 150 to 500 per ml. The increase was gradual from 2.1 to 3.4 log cycle between 0-14 days of storage. The major commercial spoilage risk with low fat spreads was that of moulds, particularly by the species of *Penicillium* and *Cladosporium*, which grow under storage conditions. The development of yeast and moulds on the product surface causes discoloration and flavour problems, also some species of mould can be infectious and can elicit allergic reactions. Recontamination during packaging would often result in the growth of yeast and moulds in the products. Psychrotrophic bacteria, which can grow at refrigerated temperature, are usually responsible for spoilage of the spread. Psychrotrophic counts in spreads after 4 weeks of storage at 7.2°C, may ranged from 10 to 130 per ml.

Factors Affecting Shelf life of Table Spreads

Various factors influences the spoilage and thereby the shelf life of the fat spreads, they are:-

i. ***Moisture content*** : Water activity of any food system is one of the important factor affecting shelf life. In general the moisture content of table spreads varies from 30-50% and consequently the shelf life is shorter. The concept of water activity and its effect on microbial growth is well known. Bacteria usually require higher moisture activity while moulds can grow at lower water activity.

ii. ***Process treatment*** : Oil-in-water emulsion are generally considered to have poor shelf life as compared to water-in-oil emulsion. The bacteriological quality of water-in-oil emulsion is closely related to the size of serum droplet dispersed in continuous phase. Droplets of less than 10 micron in diameter would not support th growth of bacteria. Rapid spoilage occurs when the droplet size exceeds 50 micron. Spreads having droplet size in the range of 3-10 micron have excellent shelf life.

iii. ***Type of ingredients*** : Dispersion of serum in the fat phase is influenced by the level of fat in the spread. It appears that serum in 38.8% fat spread is more finally dispersed than in 30% fat spread. Finer serum dispersion permits satisfactory keeping quality.

iv. ***Salt content*** : Addition of common salt generally improves flavour acceptability of the spreads. In addition it also acts as preservative by suppressing growth of bacteria and fungi when added at the rate of 1.0-1.5%.

v. ***pH of the product*** : Low pH generally restrict growth of micro-organisms. Un-dissociated acid are primarily responsible for the preservative effect and therefore lower the pH, greater is the inhibitory action on bacterial growth. In heat processed spreads low pH would not only check proliferation of spoilage microbes but also retard growth of certain toxin producing anaerobes.

vi. ***Temperature of storage*** : Table spreads and similar products require lower temperature of storage. At ambient temperatures these products do not have appreciable shelf stability. Table spreads have shelf life of 10-12 days at 30ºC, 28-30 days at 20ºC and 60-90 days at 4º-6ºC.

vii. ***Preservative level*** : Shelf life of table spreads can be enhaced by addition of preservatives. Addition of 0.1% sorbic acid suppresses the microbial growth and helps to enhance shelf life of fat spread by another 10 days.

Factors Influencing Spreadability

Spreadability is one of the most highly regarded attributes of spreads. This is probably the most important attribute for table margarines and spreads. To the consumer, spreadability is the ease with which the margarine can be applied in a thin, even layer on bread. To produce a spreadable margarine, there should be three conditions to meet while formulating product.

i. The liquid and solid phases of oils must co-exist.

ii. The solid crystals must be sufficient in numbers and finely dispersed throughout the entire mass of margarine and solid crystals must be effectively held together in the crystal matrix by internal cohesive force to prevent the entrapped liquid from seeping away.

iii. The proper proportions of solid and liquid fat should be present at a certain temperature and the crystals should melt at below body temperature.

Thus, spreadability is influenced by solid fat content (SFC) and polymorphic form of fat in spreads.

Solid fat content or solid fat index : Solid fat content (SFC) is an important property of an oil or fat, and is the ratio of the solid to the total phase at a particular temperature. This phenomenon is especially important in case of margarine. A product with 10-20% SFC at the serving temperature will have good spreadability.

Polymorphic form : Polymorphic forms are the different crystalline structures of the same chemical composition. It is the ability of fat to exist in different crystal forms. Tri-acyl glycerol can crystallize in different polymorphs with the four major forms, they are sub-α, α, β' and β. Transformation from one polymorph to another can occur in the solid state without melting. The change is from the lowest to the highest melting point, that is, from α to β' and β' to β form or towards the more stable form (Nawar 1985). The β'-crystal polymorph occurs as single needle-shaped crystals about 5–7 μm long, while the β-crystal polymorph is 20-30μm long. The smaller the crystal size is desirable for smoother product, while bigger crystals impart coarse, grainy and brittle texture to the product.

Suggested Readings

Deshpande, D. and Thompkinson, D.K. (2000). Sensory Quality of Table Spread. Processed Food Industry, 3 (8):14-20.

Deshpande, D. and Thompkinson, D.K. (2000). Table spreads – A Review. Ind.J.Dairy Sci., LIII (3): 154-168.

Deshpande, D. and Thompkinson, D.K. (2001). Formulation of Table Spread from UF Retentate: Product Standardization. Processed Food Industry, 5 (1) : 20-29.

Early Ralph (1998). The Technology of Dairy Products, Second edition. PP:179-180 Blackie Academic & Professional, Thomson Science. London UK.

Miskandar, M.S., Yaakob Che Man, Yusoff, M.S.A. and Rahman, R.A. (2005). Quality of Margarine: Fats Selection and Processing Parameters. Asia Pac. J. Clin. Nutr., 14(4):387-395.

Moran, D.P.J. (1994). Fats in spredable products. In: Fats in food products (Moran, D.P.J. and Rajah, K,K. eds.) Blackie Academic and Professional, London, p.155.

Nawar, W.W. (1985). Lipids. In: Food Chemistry: 2nd revised and expended ed. New York: Marcel Dekker Inc; 139-245.

Suman Kharb and Thompkinson, D.K. (2007). Low fat spread having functional attributes. Poster presentation at 7th Panborn Sensory Sci. Symposium, Minnepolis, USA (Abst. No. PAANG2007-132).

Suman Kharb (2007). Formulation of table spread with added functional ingredients. Ph.D. thesis submitted to NDRI Deemed University, Karnal, Haryana.

6

Ghee and Butter Oil

Introduction

Ghee is the pure clarified butter fat prepared chiefly from cream and/or *desi* butter (*Makhan*) to which no colouring matter is added. Ghee manufacture has great significance and relevance to Indian masses and the dairy industry. Ghee is a very popular product since ancient time and has greater demand during festival and other ceremonial functions where use of ghee in food has been considered to delicacy due to its pleasing flavour and aroma. There are sufficient recorded evidence to prove that the manufacture of ghee originated from India and has been used extensively for religious and dietary purposes since Vedic times. Presently about 28% of total milk production is utilized for manufacture of about 1 million tones of ghee per annum. It is the traditional product with an established market. Cow *ghee* is golden yellow in colour, and is attributed unique therapeutic value. The colour of buffalo ghee is greenish yellow due to presence of pigments called *billirubin* and *billiverdin*. *Ghee* is characterized by its pleasant, cooked and rich flavour. The preferred texture is of larger uniform size from grains having non-greasy consistency. Various factors effect the flavour development in ghee at different levels like house hold, trading centers and organized dairies in India. These factors are:-

1. Simple technology and low cost
2. Longer shelf life
3. No special storage requirements

4. Best way to salvage substandard and return milk through fat recovery
5. Several usage – Religious rites, cooking/frying medium, direct dressing of foods

Necessity for production of ghee

India, being a tropical country, experience wider variations in ambient temperature from region to region and from season to season. It is very difficult to provide a cold chain to protect perishable products like milk, cream and butter for longer time as this exercise involves additional investment and expenditure. Thus any simple, convenient and affordable process to preserve milk fat would favor the milk producers and processors to a greater extent.

Milk producers, in India mainly refer to small and marginal farmers, experience great difficulty to preserve milk whenever excess milk is left with them. Conversion of milk to *dahi* and then from *dahi* to ghee was found to be the only affordable and convenient way to preserve milk fat at household level due to limited resources availability and due to longer shelf life of ghee at ambient temperature. In industry also, the best ways to salvage substandard and returned market milk or *dahi* (especially leaked pouches) is separation of fat from these sources and convert this fat into ghee.

Ghee is a very popular product since ancient time and have greater demand during festival and other ceremonial functions wherein use of ghee in food preparation has been considered to be delicacy due to its pleasing flavour and aroma. Ghee has a market demand of more than one million ton per annum in India (FAO 2011), to meet this huge demand and also involvement of simple technology to produce ghee attracts the milk processor to have ghee making plant of variable capacity.

Definition

According to FSSAI-2011, ghee means the pure heat clarified fat derived solely from milk or curd or from desi (cooking) butter or from cream to which no colouring matter or preservative has been added.

Table: 6.1: Standards for ghee state wise in India (FSSAI-2011)

Sl. No.	Name of the State / Union Territory	Butyro-Refractometer reading at 40°C	Minimum Reichert Value	Percentage of	
				FFA as oleic acid (max.)	Moisture (Max.)
1.	Andhra Pradesh	40.0 to 43.0	24	3	0.5
2.	Andaman & Nicobar Islands	40.0 to 43.0	24	3	0.5
3.	Arunachal Pradesh	41.0 to 44.0	26	3	0.5
4.	Assam	40.0 to 43.0	26	3	0.5
5.	Bihar	40.0 to 43.0	28	3	0.5
6.	Chandigarh	40.0 to 43.0	28	3	0.5
7.	Chattisgarh	40.0 to 44.0	26	3	0.5
8.	Dadra and Nagar haveli	40.0 to 43.0	24	3	0.5
9.	Delhi	40.0 to 43.0	28	3	0.5
10.	Goa	40.0 to 43.0	26	3	0.5
11.	Daman & Diu	40.0 to 43.5	24	3	0.5
12.	Gujarat				
12a.	Areas other than cotton tract areas	40.0 to 43.5	24	3	0.5
12b.	Cotton tract areas	41.5 to 45.0	21	3	0.5
13.	Haryana				
13a.	Areas other than cotton tract areas	40.0 to 43.0	28	3	0.5
13b.	Cotton tract areas	40.0 to 43.0	26	3	0.5
14.	Himachal Pradesh	40.0 to 43.0	26	3	0.5
15.	Jammu & Kashmir	40.0 to 43.0	26	3	0.5
16.	Jharkhand	40.0 to 43.0	28	3	0.5
17.	Karnataka			3	0.5
17a.	Areas other than Belgaum district	40.0 to 43.0	24	3	0.5
17b.	Belgaum district	40.0 to 44.0	26	3	0.5
18.	Kerala	40.0 to 43.0	26	3	0.5
19.	Lakshwadeep	40.0 to 43.0	26	3	0.5
20.	Madhya Pradesh				
20a.	Areas other than cotton tract areas	40.0 to 43.0	26	3	0.5
20b.	Cotton tract areas	41.5 to 45.0	21	3	0.5
21.	Maharashtra				
21a.	Areas other than cotton tract areas	40.0 to 43.0	26	3	0.5
21b.	Cotton tract areas	41.5 to 45.0	21	3	0.5
22.	Manipur	40.0 to 43.0	26	3	0.5
23.	Meghalya	40.0 to 43.0	26	3	0.5
24.	Mizoram	40.0 to 43.0	26	3	0.5

Contd.

Contd. Table 6.1

Sl. No.	Name of the State / Union Territory	Butyro-Refractometer reading at 40°C	Minimum Reichert Value	Percentage of	
				FFA as oleic acid (max.)	Moisture (Max.)
25.	Nagaland	40.0 to 43.0	26	3	0.5
26.	Odisha	40.0 to 43.0	26	3	0.5
27.	Puducherry	40.0 to 44.0	26	3	0.5
28.	Punjab	40.0 to 43.0	28	3	0.5
29.	Rajasthan				
29a.	Areas other than Jodhpur District	40.0 to 43.0	26	3	0.5
29b.	Jodhpur District	41.5 to 45.0	21	3	0.5
30.	Tamil Nadu	41.0 to 44.0	24	3	0.5
31.	Tripura	40.0 to 43.0	26	3	0.5
32.	Uttar Pradesh	40.0 to 43.0	26	3	0.5
33.	Uttarakhand	40.0 to 43.0	26	3	0.5
34.	West Bengal				
34a.	Areas other than Bishnupur sub division	40.0 to 43.0	28	3	0.5
34b.	Bishnupur sub division	41.5 to 45.0	21	3	0.5
34.	Sikkim	40.0 to 43.0	28	3	0.5

Product Description and Chemical Composition of Ghee

Ghee could be in liquid, semisolid and some time in solid state based on type of fat (liquid vs solid) and the storage temperature. Ghee made from buffalo milk is whitish with greenish tinge and that of cow milk is golden yellow colour. It is usually prepared form cow milk, buffalo milk or mixed milk.

Composition

Ghee majorly constitute of milk lipids and is the richest source of milk fat of all Indian Dairy products. The constitutent of ghee tend to vary with the method of manufacture. Chemically ghee is a complex lipid of glycerides (majorly triglycerides – 97 to 98%), small amount of di- and mono-glycerides and traces of free fatty acids, phospholipids, sterols, sterol esters, fat soluble vitamins, carbonyls, hydrocarbons, carotenoids, (only in ghee derived from cow milk). Detailed chemical composition of cow milk ghee and buffalo milk ghee is given below.

Table 6.2: Chemical composition of ghee

Constituents	Cow milk ghee	Buffalo milk ghee
Fat (%)	99 to 99.5	
Moisture (%)	Not more than 0.5	
Carotene (mg/g)	3.2-7.4	-
Vitamin A (IU/g)	19-34	17-38
Cholesterol (mg/100g)	302 – 362	209 – 312
Tocopherol (mg/g)	26 – 48	18 – 31
Free fatty acid (%)	Max. 2.8	

Source: Wadhwa, 2002.

The fatty acid may be saturated or unsaturated and usually contains an even number of carbon atoms. Fatty acid composition of buffalo milk ghee also varies from cow milk ghee. The amount of butyric acid is significantly higher in buffalo milk ghee than in cow milk ghee. The levels of short chain fatty acids from caproic acid to myristic acid are significantly higher in cow milk ghee than buffalo milk ghee where as levels of palmitic acids and stearic acids are higher in buffalo milk ghee than in cow milk ghee. Major fatty acids distribution in cow milk fat and buffalo milk fat is given below.

Table 6.3: BIS requirements for ghee

Product	Fat (% min)	Moisture (% min)	BR reading (40°C)	RM value† (min)	FFA (%)	PV (meq/kg fat) max.
Ghee	99.50	0.50	40-45	21-24	0.30	0.80

† 21 for Gujarat and 24 for imported butter oil

Methods of Ghee Making

The principle involved in ghee preparation includes concentration of milk fat in the form of cream or butter, followed by heat clarification of fat rich milk portion and thus reducing the amount of water to less than 0.5%. The curd content is then removed as ghee residue by filtration from clarified fat.

There are five methods of ghee making:

1. Desi or Indigenous Method
2. Direct Cream Method
3. Creamery Butter Method
4. Pre-stratification Method
5. Continuous Method

Desi or Indigenous Method

The *desi* method accounts for the bulk of *ghee* produced in India. This was the practice from age-old days in rural areas where excessive milk will be cultured and kept for overnight for fermentation. Resultant curd was churned using hand driven wooden beaters to separate the milk fat in the form of desi butter. In this method, *dahi* is prepared by culturing lukewarm milk with 2 percent of the previous day's butter-milk or *dahi.* The dahi is then churned in earthen vessels by wooden churners for 20 to 30 minutes, and the butter grains so formed are removed from the paddle and from the surface of the buttermilk by hand. The butter thus obtained is then heated over a medium and steady fire till the moisture is removed. *Ghee* produced at different places and different conditions vary in quality. It is refined by heating in large pans at 90° to 110°C, the product being allowed to settle for 2 to 5 hours after removing the scum formed at the top. The clear *ghee* is packed and stored in tins in a cool place for proper crystallization or grain formation. The recovery of the fat is about 60 to 80 percent of the total fat content in butter.

Some follow slightly different method wherein milk is heated continuously to about 80⁰C, the malai (creamy layer) that forms over the surface was collected manually. this malai is then churned to get the desi butter. After collection of desi butter over a period of time, this butter is melted in a metal pan or earthenware vessel on an open fire. Extent of frothing is an index to judge when to terminate heating. Heating should be stop when sudden foaming appears and leave the contents undisturbed after heating. Curd particles starts settling down over a period of time and decant the clear fat carefully. In this method it is possible to achieve only 75-85% fat recovery.

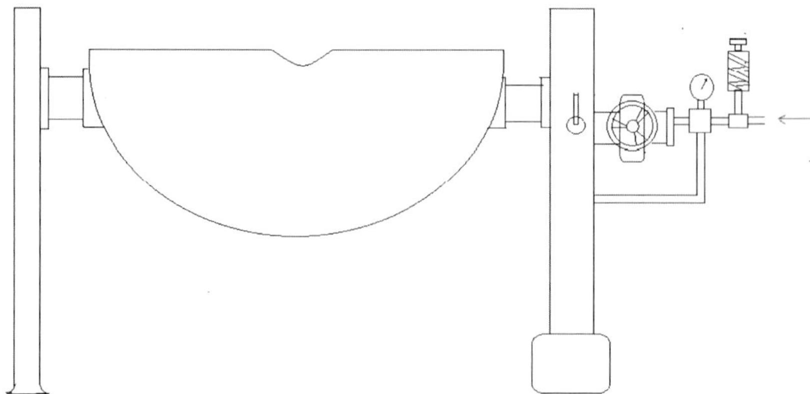

Fig. 6.1: Tilting type ghee kettle

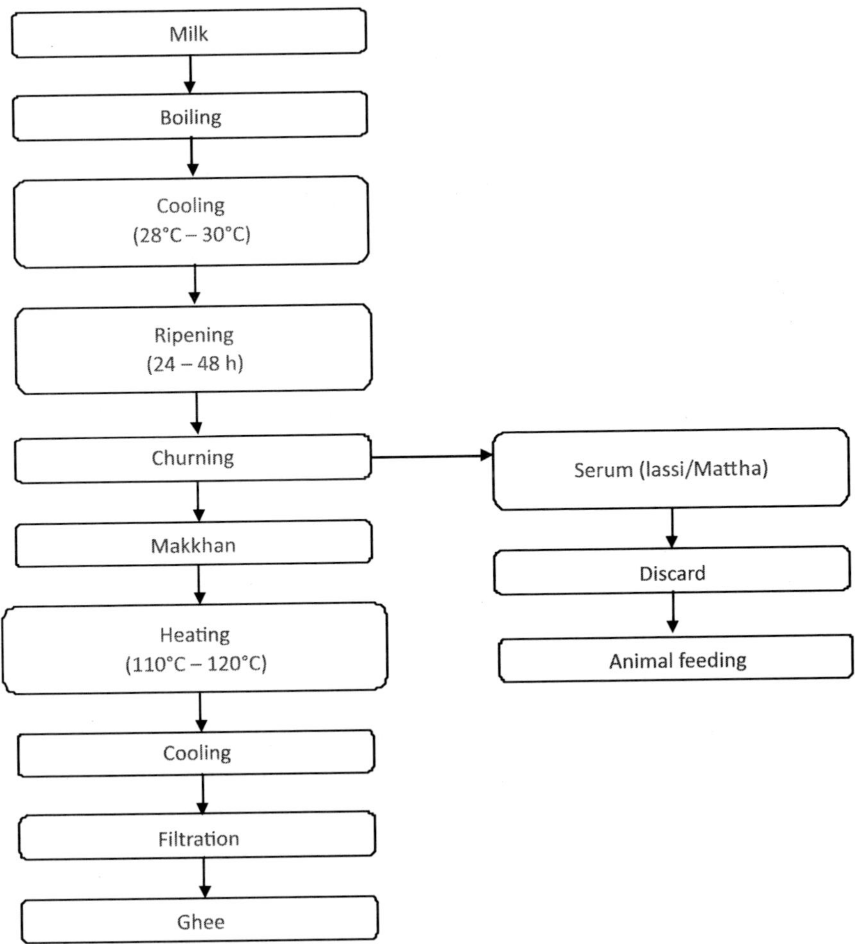

Fig. 6.2: Desi method of ghee making

Creamery Butter Method

The creamery method of making *ghee* is in vogue mainly in organised sector of dairies. This is the standard method adopted in most of the organized dairies. Unsalted or white butter is used as raw material. The cream is first converted to unsalted butter which is then melted in a butter melter at 80° C. The molten butter is then pumped into ghee boiler/kettle or pan for final heating. Ghee boiler/kettle is generally a double jacketed equipment of various capacities where steam is used as a heating media. During the heating process, when the temperature is less than 100° C, frothing starts with scum formation at the surface. This scum is removed with perforated ladle. The moisture is constantly driven off and as the temperature crosses 100° C mark; a second foaming appears with effervescence and appearance of final air bubbles with crackling sound. At this stage the ghee residue turns to golden brown colour. There is sudden rice in temperature and hence heating has to be stopped to avoid overheating. Final heating temperature is adjusted to about 114±2° C. To get the cooked flavour, heating beyond this temperature is also being in practice A typical aroma of ghee is also noticed at this stage. The contents are allowed to cool slowly. When temperature reaches down to 75-80° C, the ghee is passed through a filter cloth or an oil separator to remove residues. The clarified ghee is then packed in suitable containers and stored in granulation chamber (16-20° C) for 7-10 day before merchandising. The ghee prepared from creamery butter has a better keeping quality but lacks the flavor of ghee as compared to ghee prepared from *desi* method. Because of the lower curd content of creamery butter, the loss of fat in ghee residue is lower and the recovery of butterfat is about 90-96 percent.

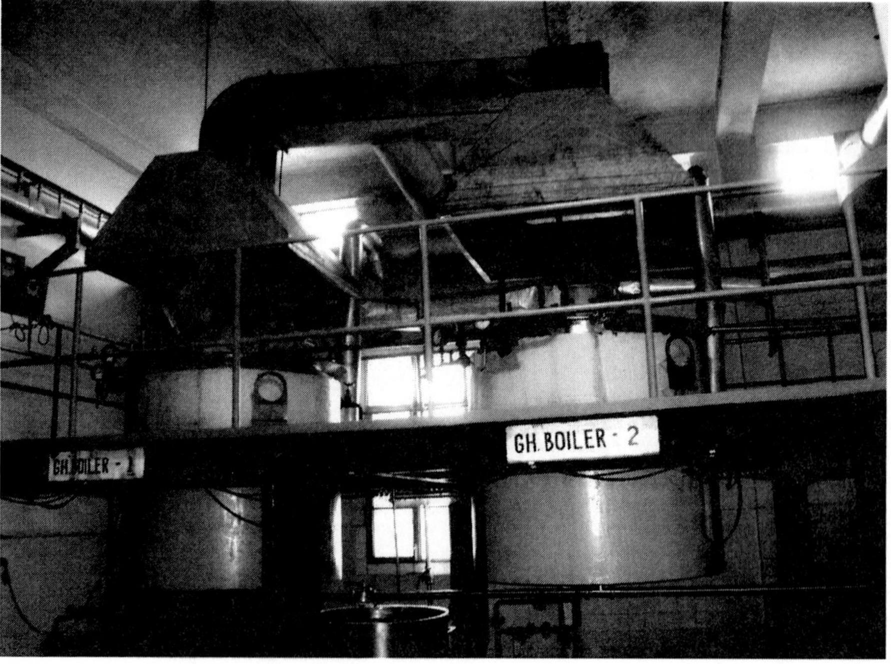

Fig. 6.3: Ghee boiler

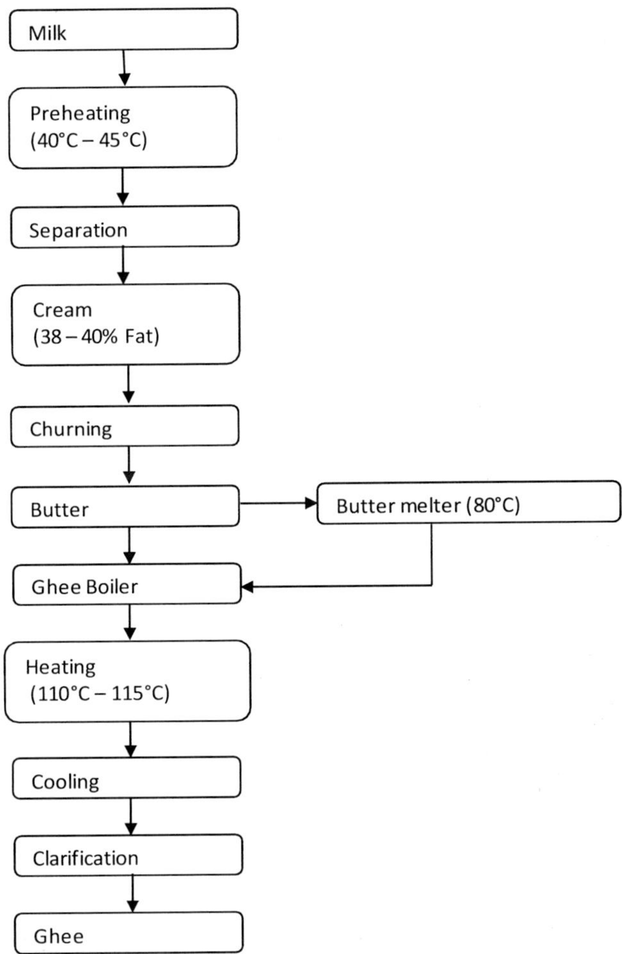

Fig. 6.4: Creamery butter method of ghee manufacture

Direct Cream Method

Ghee may also be prepared directly by boiling fresh cream or cultured cream. This method involves separation of cream of 60 to 70% fat from milk by centrifugation process. The improved method for the manufacture of ghee directly from cream is to re-separate it after diluting it with water to the original volume of milk.

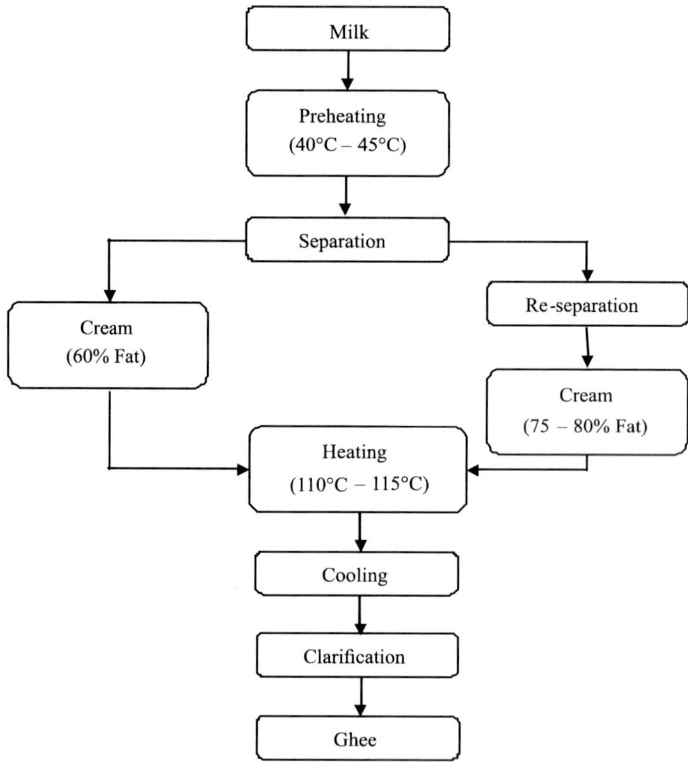

Fig. 6.5: Direct Cream Method

This reduces the curd content of cream and therefore loss of butter fat in ghee residue is less. Cream is heated to 110°C to 115°C in a stainless steel, jacketed ghee kettle. Ghee kettle is usually fitted with an agitator, steam control knob, pressure and temperature gauges. A movable hollow stainless tube centrally bored for emptying out the contents or alternatively provision can be made for tilting device to decant the ghee. Heating is discontinued as soon as the colour of the ghee residue turns to golden yellow or light brown. During the heating process, plenty of effervescence accompanied by a crackling sound is observed in the preliminary stages of boiling but both gradually subsides as soon as the moisture is evaporated. When almost all the moisture is evaporated, the temperature of the liquid medium suddenly spurts up and utmost care has to be exercised at this stage to control the heating. The end point is indicated by the appearance of second effervescence, which is subtler than the first one accompanied by the browning of curd particles. At this stage the typical ghee flavour emanates and this indicates that the final stage in the preparation of ghee. The recovery of fat in this method is 80 to 85 percent.

A major advantage of this method is there is no need for butter production prior to manufacturing of ghee. But, it has several limitations as listed below.

i. It takes longer heating time to evaporate the moisture.

ii. The amount of ghee residue produced during this method is higher; hence, there is a loss of 4 to 6 percent of butter fat in the ghee residue. Therefore, it is recommended to use 70 to 80 percent fat cream to minimize both fat loss and steam consumption.

iii. The higher amount of serum solids in the cream may also produce a highly caramelized flavour in the ghee.

Pre-stratification Method

This method consists of holding the molten butter undisturbed for a period of 30-50 minutes in a specially designed tank having a faucet fitted at the bottom of the tank. The process allows the molten mixture to separate out into three different layers based on density of constituents. The bottom layer of buttermilk solids consists of 80% of moisture and 70% of solids-not-fat contained in butter. The middle layer consists of liquid fat where as a thin top layer has small amount of serum. After the set period of time, the bottom layer is removed by opening the faucet and discarded.

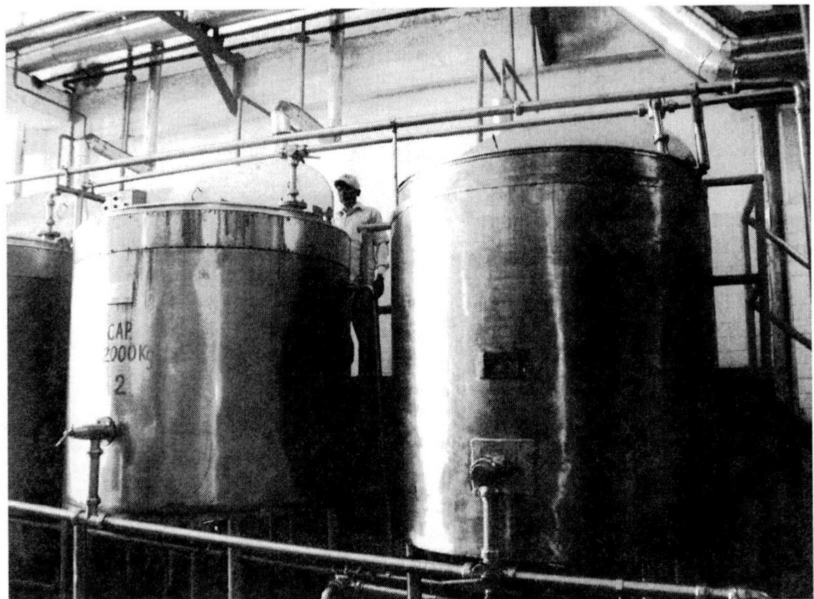

Fig. 6.6: Pre-stratification tank

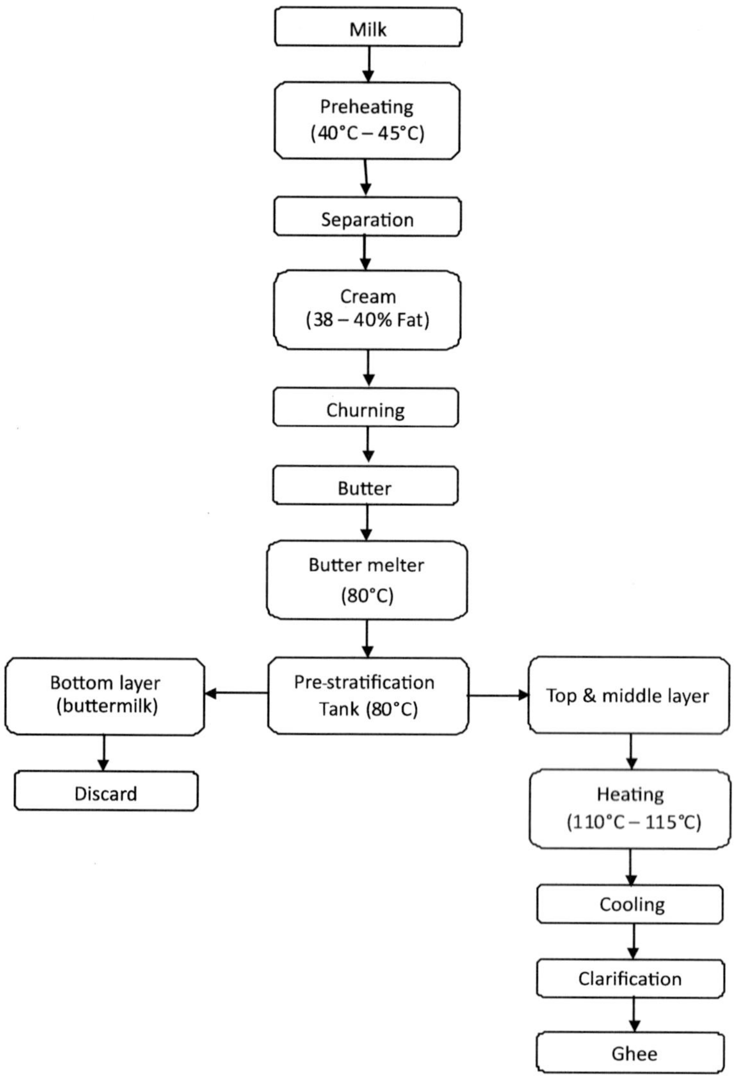

Fig. 6.7: Pre-stratification method of ghee making

The rest of the contents are heated to 110° C to 115° C to free it completely from moisture and to precipitate small amount of remaining curd. This step is necessary to develop characteristic ghee flavour. The ghee thus prepared is allowed to cool before clarification. The clarified ghee is then packed and stored in granulation chamber and finally stored at room temperature. The process permit production of milder flavour ghee, since most of the curd content is removed in the bottom layer before final clarification temperature is reached.

This method is economical from the point of fuel consumption to the extent of 35 to 50 percent. It saves time and consequently labor costs to the extent of about 45 percent, besides yielding a product which is superior in keeping quality.

There are several advantages of this method as listed below.

i. Removal of buttermilk (bottom layer) eliminates prolonged heating for evaporation of the moisture.

ii. Formation of significantly low quantity of ghee residue, absorbing low quantity of fat, hence minimizes fat loss with ghee residue.

iii. Ghee prepared by this method has lower free fatty acid and acidity.

Continuous Method

Increasing demand of ghee in Indian market triggers dairy industry to adapt continuous ghee manufacturing method. This method also assures uniform quality and greater economy of ghee production on an industrial scale. The continuous method of ghee production has several advantages like,

i. Contamination by handlers is nil or negligible.

ii. No foaming of the product during production

iii. It has better control on quality of the product.

iv. At any point of time, continuous method holds small volume, hence no chance for whole batch getting rejected.

v. Complete plant can be connected with CIP lines.

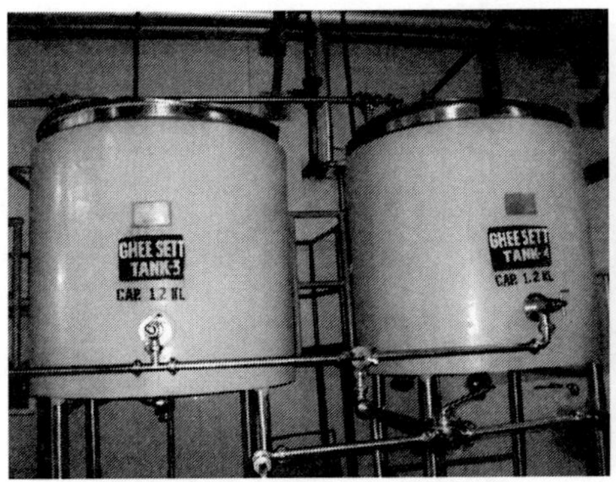

Fig. 6.8: Ghee settling tank

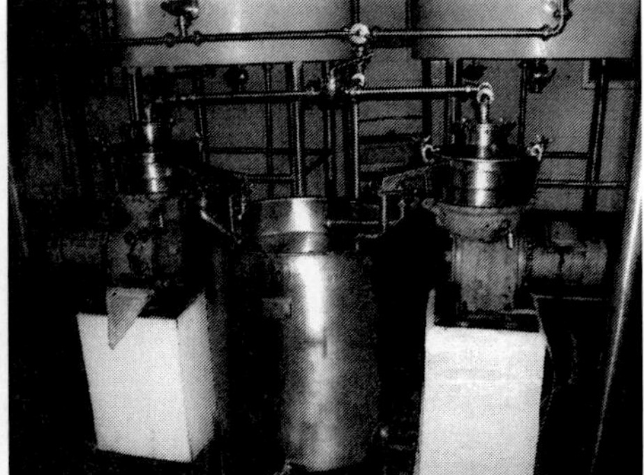

Fig. 6.9: Ghee clarifier

The continuous process also overcomes the limitations associated with batch process in terms of capacity of related equipments which are unsuitable for large volume of production, high energy requirement, enhance processing losses, spillage on floors of processing and packaging areas and difficulty in adapting CIP cleaning system.

A continuous process of ghee preparation has been developed by National Dairy Research Institute, Karnal. The process consists of melting butter in a butter melter using steam to a temperature of 90-95°C. This molten butter is then pumped through three stage thin film scrapped surface heat exchanger (TFSSHE). Each stage is connected with variable frequency drive (VFD) agitating system. During first and second stage of processing the agitation level is maintained at higher speed (up to 175 rpm) for quick moisture evaporation. During last stage of processing (third stage) the agitation speed is lowered to around 20 rpm. The steam pressure, throughout the process is maintained at 1-3kg/cm^2 at each stage of heating. Provision is also made to recirculate the product from third stage to first stage which helps to reach temperature as high as 124°C. However, ghee with better texture and flavour was obtained at a temperature of 121°C and its corresponding moisture content was 0.192%.

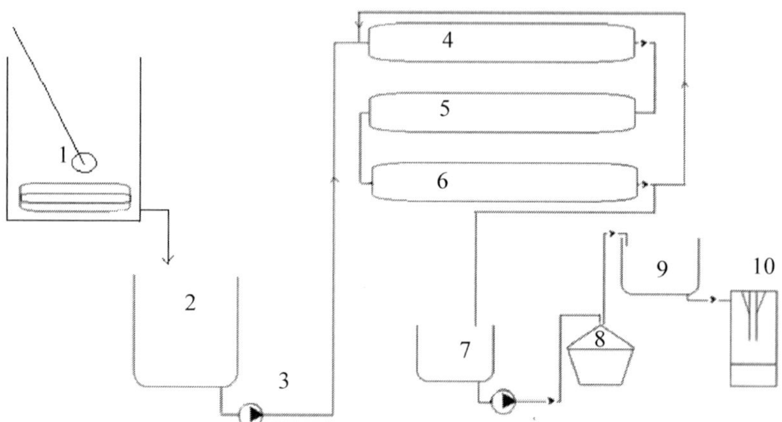

1. Butter Melter
2. Balance Tank
3. Feed Pump
4. First stage TFSSHE
5. Second stage TFSSHE
6. Third stage TFSSHE
7. Storage tank
8. Clarifier
9. Over-head tank
10. Packaging unit

Fig. 6.10: Schematic diagram of continuous ghee making equipment

Efficiency of Methods

The efficiency of various method of ghee manufacture may differ in terms of fat recovery and energy requirements. The total fat recovery from indigenous method is the lowest while energy requirement is maximum. In contrast the total fat recovery is highest in creamery butter method while the energy requirement is lowest in case of creamery butter method. Energy requirements are lowest in case of pre-stratification method for ghee making.

Table 6.4: Fat recovery and energy requirements of different methods

Methods	Fat recovery (%)	Energy requirement (Kcal/kg)
Indigenous	80 – 85 %	1710
Direct cream	88 – 92 %	1325
Creamery butter	90 – 95 %	414
Pre-stratification	92 – 97 %	270
Continuous	94 – 98 %	245

Source : From different sources

Although the recovery of fat from various methods of ghee making is in the range of 88 -98% (as shown in above table), Nevertheless, appreciable amount of fat still goes in ghee residue. This is true specially in case of direct cream method of ghee making. This fat can be recovered by treating the ghee residue with hot water. Generally in commercial dairies the ghee residue obtained is transferred into the fat recovery tank which is then filled with hot water and allowed to stand over night. The fat,being lighter in density and immisible in water, rise to the top of water layer. This is then collected and re-heated to recover fat.

Granulation and Cooling of Ghee

Ghee is one of the highly priced dietary fat in India. The Indian consumer is willing to pay a high price for this food article due to its pleasant aroma and specific texture which cannot be duplicated by any other fat. Physical properties of milk fat have profound influence on sensory attributes, in particular, texture of fat rich dairy products. In addition to aroma/flavour of ghee, its texture in terms of number and size of fat granules is an important criterion in judging the quality of ghee. Presence of uniform large grains with very little liquid fat is desirable characteristic. Ghee with greasy or waxy texture is not liked by consumers and therefore granulation is an important criterion of quality.

The presence of saturated and unsaturated straight chain fatty acids in milk fat imparts a unique physical spectrum of characteristics in terms of crystallization behavior and melting point range. The wide melting range of milk fat helps in selective crystallization phenomenon in clarified butter fat. The process chiefly depends on cooling process. The texture of ghee depends on source of fat, method of manufacture, clarification temperature, rate of cooling and a storage temperature.. Granular ghee develops lesser degree of rancidity as compare to ghee having fat in liquid state. If ghee is cooled rapidly large number of very fine crystals are formed consisting of a mixture of high and low melting points such ghee develops smooth grease like texture. In contrast slow cooling of ghee leads to formation of few crystals consisting of high melting point. With the progress of cooling more and more fat solidify leading to formation of large crystals suspended liquid fat. The granulation of ghee is a complex phenomenon. The major constituent of milk fat is triglycerides with different physical and chemical properties. It is primarily due to different melting points of triglycerides. The higher melting point saturated fatty acids, especially palmitic acid and stearic acid have greater control on granulation. Thus buffalo milk ghee show predominant granulation than cow milk ghee. When the molten fat is cooled the intermolecular forces draw the triglycerides closure with a parallel ordering of fatty acids chains. This is the first step towards crystallization process with formation of crystal nuclei due to molecular gathering. As the temperature falls the rate of nucleation increases until it reaches maximum. The growth of crystal nuclei takes place by deposition of successive layers on an already formed crystal surface. In absence of stirring the solidified fat tends to flocculate into a network held together by forces of attraction. As crystallization advances almost all of remaining liquid phase is bound into the network. The mass appears as a complete solid although it does consist of certain amount of liquid fat. For better granulation, ghee should be slowly cooled to 28°C in 2-3 hours time.

Various factors influence the grain formation in ghee, among them major ones are listed in Table 6.5.

Table 6.5: Factors affecting the granulation in ghee

S.No.	Factor	Effect on granulation
1.	Feed	It alters the fatty acid profile of milk fat, thus it alters the amount of saturated fat and unsaturated fat.
2.	Season	Significantly larger grains are formed in winter than in summer and monsoon.
3.	Fatty acid profile	saturated fatty acids increases the grains size whereas unsaturated fat increases the liquid portion
4.	Method of manufacture	Desi method yields good grainy texture whereas direct cream method yields greasy texture
5.	Seeding	Seeding yields needle-like grainy structure compared to spherical ones without seeding
6.	Rate of cooling	Rapid cooling yields smaller crystals, slow cooling yields bigger crystals
7.	Storage temperature	Cold storage causes development of waxy consistency
8.	Temperature of clarification	The higher temperature of clarification gives better grain size due to high phospholipids content

Preservation of Ghee

Clarified fat or ghee has much better capacity to resist elemental and microbial attack and resultant spoilage than many other milk products. When produced, packed and stored under controlled hygienic conditions, it is expected to have a shelf life of about 9 months at 21° C. the shelf life of ghee is mainly effected by degree of unsaturation of fat, storage temperature, initial acidity and moisture content of ghee, presence of oxygen and catalytic salts like iron and copper, packing conditions etc. Prolonged storage of ghee at ambient temperature may result in oxidative changes causing production of objectionable flavour, formation of toxic compounds, loss of unsaturated fatty acids, loss of nutritive value, and attractive colour. It is possible to increase the durability of ghee by adopting following practices.

Using good quality raw material : Cream or butter used for making ghee should be of good quality. Any off flavour – acidic, rancid and oxidized, present in cream or butter will be carried over to the final product. Ghee prepared by indigenous method using high acid curd, thus have shorter shelf life. Care should also be taken that cream or butter does not contain any catalytic salt at any stage of manufacture, that may start the catalytic reaction leading to spoilage of ghee during storage.

Addition of antioxidants : There are number of natural as well as synthetic antioxidants available and can be added in small quantities (ppm) as permitted legally by food safety law. These antioxidants are added for complete prevention or partial retardation of oxidation of fat (unsaturated fatty acids) during storage. Amongst the synthetic antioxidants are Butylated hydroxytoluene (BHT), Butylated hydroxyanisole (BHA), ethyl, propyl and octyl gallates and tertiary butyl hydroquinone (BHTQ) where as ascorbic acid, alpha-tocopherol, phospholipids etc are some of the natural antioxidants. The age old practice of boiling betel and curry leaves during clarification of acidic curd into ghee (indigenous method) improves the flavour, colour and shelf life of ghee.

Packaging of Ghee

Ghee has comparatively longer keeping quality. It can be stored for 6 to 12 months under ambient temperature provided it is properly filled and packaged. Exposure of ghee to light, air, water vapour and metals causes deterioration of ghee as mentioned below:

1. Sunlight	Causes light induced oxidation & associated off flavours
2. Air (Oxygen)	Causes oxidation/oxidative rancidity in ghee
3. Water Vapour	Causes hydolytic rancidity
4. Metals (Copper & Iron)	Catalyzes rancidity development

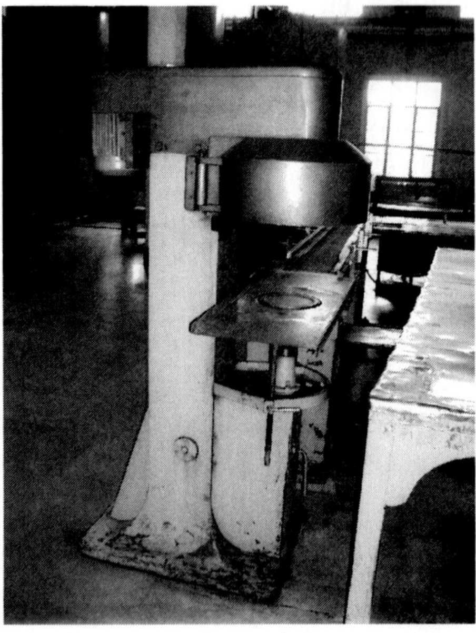

Fig. 6.11: Ghee tin packing machine

It is therefore necessary that packaging material should prevent the entry of light, air, water vapour and contact with metals. Minimum or no head space should be provided while filling and always it is better to fill the product upto the brim of the container. Ghee is generally packed in lacquered tin containers ranging from 250 g to 15 kg. It is also packed in plastic screw capped bottles ranging from 100 g to 5 kg. Recently, flexible packaging materials and self standing laminates (HDPE, PP, metalized polyester pouches) are widely being in use due to their low cost and convenience. These materials have low water vapour transmission rate. Ghee packed in flexible pouches should be placed in paper cartons containing some cushioning material to protect the pouch during transportation and rough handling. Efforts must be made to reduce oxygen content of package to minimum level by keeping lesser head space in a package. In tin container it is best to replace oxygen with nitrogen gas to prevent lipid oxidation. Since, exposure of ghee to sunlight for a long time causes oxidation and produce off flavors; therefore, it should be stored in a dark cool place, preferably at a temperature of 21-22°C. Apart from these, packaging materials should withstand wear and tear during transportation, protect against tempering and easily available at low cost. It should not allow printing ink to penetrate into the product, should not react with ghee and it should be non toxic.

Common Packaging Materials for Ghee

1. ***Tin cans*** : Tin cans are popular for bulk packing of ghee viz., 1L, 2L, 5L and 15L. These are formed by low carbon steel sheets (thickness ranging from 0.15 to 0.40mm) coated with tin (0.5 to 34g/m^2) on both sides through electro-deposition process. The cans should be sealed properly to prevent the entry of oxygen as it causes oxidation in the product during storage. It is very essential that tin cans must be coated with lacquer coating inside. Only drawback in tin cans is the cost. Higher cost renders its use and to search for cost competitive packaging material.

2. ***Glass bottles*** : Traditionally glass bottles were popular in retail packs. Glass bottles provide excellent protection to the product quality as they do not react with the food material. Following are the limitations of glass bottles.

    i. Highly fragile in nature, so there is a possibility of breakage during handling.

    ii. Comparatively heavy in weight, increases the transportation cost of the product.

iii. Secondary packaging material must provide cushioning effect to these bottles to prevent breakage during transportation, thus increasing packaging cost of the product.

3. ***Semi-rigid containers*** : In recent time, semi-rigid plastic containers are replacing tin plate containers. These are mainly made out of high density polyethylene (HDPE). The advantages of using these containers are light-weight, economical and transport-worthy. They are of several types, viz., blow moulded HDPE (high density polyethylene), PET (polyethylene terephthalate) bottles, PVC (poly vinyl chloride) bottles, lines çartons and tetra packs. Blow moulded HDPE are, available in form of bottles (200, 400g), jars (1 kg and 2 kg), and jerry cans (2kg, 5kg, and 15kg). These e semi-rigid containers have potential to explore in near future.

4. ***Flexible films/pouches/laminates*** : Flexible pouches are usually made from laminates or multi layer films of different composition and in the form of pillow pouches or self-standing pouches. Packaging ghee in pouch is cheaper compare to other modes and can be easily adaptable at commercial plant. The selection of laminate or a multi layer film is governed primarily by the compatibility of the contact layer, heat-sealing ability and heat-seal strength and shelf life required. Flexible laminate made up of PVDC/PVC/Al foil/PP (polyvinyliedene chloride/aluminium foil/polypropylene) are suitable for long-term storage of butter oil and ghee.

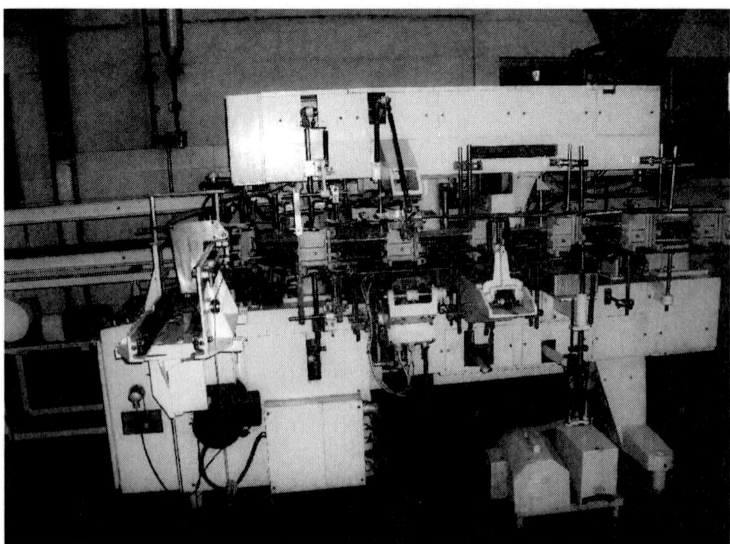

Fig. 6.12: Ghee pouch packing machine (Cekapack)

Storage of Ghee

Storage at higher temperature leads to development of oxidized flavor especially with ghee which has pronounced initial acidity. Storage at low (refrigerated) temperature imparts greasy and pasty texture in ghee although it slightly extends the shelf life by inhibiting acid development. Therefore, storage temperature of 21° C is recommended. It has shelf life of 6 months at 21° C.

Keeping Quality

It is the duration in which product is sensorily acceptable and safe for consumption. Ghee is more prone to oxidation induced changes during storage. Several factors influence the keeping quality of ghee and are listed below:

Factors Influencing Keeping Quality of Ghee

1. Temperature of storage: Higher the temperature of storage, lower will be the keeping quality and vice versa.
2. Initial moisture content: Higher the initial moisture content, lower will be the keeping quality and vice versa.
3. Initial acidity: Higher the initial acidity, lower the keeping quality and vice versa.
4. Exposure to metals: When ghee comes in contact with metals especially iron and copper, its keeping quality gets reduced as they catalyses the oxidation.
5. Exposure to light: Longer exposure to sunlight causes oxidation of ghee and thus reduces the shelf life.
6. Method of packaging**:** Higher amount of air-content in the head-space lowers the keeping quality and vice versa.

Yield

The yield of ghee from cream or butter is influenced by fat content of raw material. Factors which influence the yield are discussed below.

i. ***Method of production*** : The fat recovery in various methods of ghee preparation is given in table. 6.4.
ii. ***The fat content of the raw material used*** : Higher the fat content, higher will be the yield and vice versa.

iii. ***Quality of milk or cream*** : High acid milk or cream results in higher fat losses through ghee residue thus it reduces the yield.

iv. ***Fat recovery from ghee residue*** : Extraction of as much as fat from ghee residue improves the yield. It is possible to extract the fat from ghee residue by dissolving ghee residue in hot water followed by filtration and centrifugation and this extracted fat can be added back to cream or butter melter.

Ghee Composition and Changes During Manufacture

Ghee majorly constitute of milk lipids and richest source of milk fat of all Indian Dairy products. The constituents of ghee tend to vary with the method of its manufacture. Chemically ghee is a complete lipid of glycerides, 97-98% triglycerides. Small amount of di-and mono-glycerides also present in traces. Also cow milk ghee is different from buffalo milk ghee in terms of its composition (Table 6.2). Fatty acid composition of buffalo milk ghee also varies from cow milk ghee. The amount of butyric acid is significantly higher in buffalo than in cow ghee. The levels of short chain fatty acids caproic to myristic are significantly higher in cow than buffalo ghee where as levels of palmitic and steoric are higher in buffalo than in cow ghee. Major fatty acid types in buffalo and cow milk fat is given in (Table 1.11).

Table 6.6: Saponifiable/Unsaponifiable constituents of Ghee

Constituents	Buffalo ghee	Cow ghee
Saponifiable (%)		
Short chain	45.3	37.6
Long chain	54.7	62.4
Tri-saturated	40.7	39.0
High melting	8.7	4.9
Di-glycerides	4.5	4.3
Mono-glycerides	0.60	0.70
Un-saponifiable		
Total cholesterol (mg%)	275.00	330.00
Lanosterol (µg/g)	8.25	9.32
Squalene (µg/g)	62.40	59.20
Carotene (µg/g)	0.00	7.20
Vitamin A (µg/g)	9.50	9.20
Vitamin E (µg/g)	26.40	30.50
Ubiquinone (µg/g)	6.50	5.00

Source: Sharma, 1981

Colour, Flavour and Texture of Ghee

Colour : Ghee made from buffalo milk has white (lack of carotenoids) with greenish tinge in colour and ghee made from cow milk is golden yellow in colour due to presence of carotenoids. Colour development and granulation also happens during clarification for the subsequent packaging of ghee The characteristic colour of buffalo fat has been attributed to tetrapyrozole pigments and they are biliverdin and bilivubin.

Flavour : Ghee has characteristic pleasant, nutty, slightly cooked or caramelized sweet flavour. Flavour formation in ghee happens during fermentation of cream and during clarification process. Majorly three classes of compounds are identified as flavour compounds in ghee. They are carbonyls, lactones and free fatty acids. The flavour profile is affected by method of preparation, temperature of clarification and storage period.

Flavour components are formed during ghee preparation because of the heat effect on the unfermented residue as well on fermented metabolic products (formed during ripening process) and also due to heat interaction between the native carbohydrates and protein system of cream. Cream constituents like lactose, citrate and glucose were responsible for the increase in ghee flavour components. Flavour in ghee is the result of four different mechanisms, they are:

1.	Hydrolysis	This leads to formation of free fatty acids
2.	Oxidation	Leads to release of saturated and unsaturated aldehydes, ketones, alcohols and hydrocarbons
3.	Decarboxylation	Leads to formation of alkan-2-Ones
4.	Dehydration and lactonization	Leads to formation of lactones

Carbonyls : The carbonyl compounds are the major constituents which are responsible for the flavour of ghee. Aldehydes, ketones, low molecular weight acids, oxy acids etc., are belong to carbonyl group. Though some of the carbonyl compounds derived from milk, ripened cream and some are generated during processing. The quantity of carbonyls is directly proportional to the temperature of clarification. The head space and volatile carbonyl content of fresh desi cow ghee (0.035μM/g) is higher than that of buffalo ghee (0.027μM/g). However, total carbonyl content of fresh *desi* buffalo ghee (8.64μM/g) is higher than that of cow ghee (7.2μM/g) (carbonyl content found to increase during storage.

Lactones : The lactones contribute coconut-like aroma which is associated with characteristic flavour of ghee. δ-lactones are major ones in lactones and responsible for volatile flavour of ghee. It was reported that levels δ-lactones plus δ-lactones and total lactones were higher in buffalo milk ghee than cow milk ghee. The preparation method also affects the lactones content of ghee. The levels of δ-lactones plus y-lactones were higher in ghee prepared form direct cream method (cow milk ghee 27.21ppm, buffalo milk ghee 29.75ppm) than ghee prepared from creamery butter (cow milk ghee 19.66ppm, buffalo milk ghee 25.11ppm) or *desi* (cow milk ghee 17.43ppm, buffalo milk ghee 23.45µg/g) methods (Wadwa and Jain 1985). The lactose level in butter (12 ppm) increased 1.9, 2.4, 2.8 and 3.0 fold on clarifying at 110°C, 120°C, 140° C and 180° C respectively. Heat clarification of butter at 100-120°C doubles the lactones level from butter. The lactones level in ghee showed a significant rise on storage.

Free fatty acids (FFA): FFA contribute majorly for rancid or off flavour, however some of them are responsible for ghee flavour especially short and medium chain fatty acids (C_6 to C_{10}). FFA are higher in cow ghee (5-12.3mg/g) than buffalo ghee (5.8-7.6 mg/g). FFA content of ghee also varies depending on the method of preparation, it was reported that *desi* ghee (7.6-12.3mg/g) has highest FFA than creamery butter (6.0-7.3mg/g) and direct cream method (5.8 -7.3mg/g) of ghee preparation.

Texture

Under ambient storage, ghee crystallizes into three distinct fractions or layers, (i) oily (ii) granular semi-solid at the bottom and (iii) hard flakes portion floating on the surface and sticking to the sides of the container.

Layer formation in ghee could be prevented by storing it at 18°C-20°C immediately after preparation. Ghee thus solidified could subsequently be stored at higher temperature without formation of layer. The liquid portion of ghee varies with storage temperature, shape and size of container, repeated heating and agitation, ripening of cream/butter, storage and handling, external seeding etc.

Flavour Preferences for Ghee

A perfect ghee flavour is characterized by multiple sensory perceptions. The consumer always look for the most desireable flavour, texture , colour, freshness and wholesomeness. The perception of flavour comes from the previous experience. Consumers are ready to pay premium prize for the product they like the most. Ghee made by desi method is preferd by people of Uttar Pradesh,

Delhi and Rajasthan because of its typical flavour and texture. Possibily high curd content of desi butter contribute to the rich flavour arising during heat clarification process. In Kolkata market slightly oxidized ghee is preferred, although in other parts of India it is considered flavour defect. There has always been regional preferences for flavour of ghee. In the Northen region of country people prefer slightly acidic and mild curdy flavour in ghee. hereas in Southern and Eastern region a slightly cooked to definitely cooked and burnt flavour is preferred. In contrast people of Western region prefer mil;d to strongly curdy flavour in their ghee. The pereference in quality is determined by the end usage of ghee.

Simulation of Ghee Flavour

The acidic and curdy flavour of ghee is because of ripening of milk to form curd, before it is converted to butter and finally to ghee. This is the usual practice followed at rural level that provides desi ghee its typical flavour that lingers for long time in the mouth. However, in commercial dairies these treatments require additional space and energy. Therefore, viability of each treatment has to be viewed from the angle of ease of operation, processing cost, handling losses, scale up feasibility, quality of resultant product and its shelf life. Simulation studies have been limited to the treatment of cream and butter. Alternatively, butter oil may be used as base for ghee making as it has longer shelf life. Various approaches that have been tried to simulate curdy flavour in factory made ghee could be:-

i) Blending of conventionally made ghee with sour milk ghee.

ii) Use of starter culture for fermenting dairy butter.

iii) Blending of butter with fresh or reconstituted sour skim milk/ butter milk/ lassi at one of the following stages – during churning or working stage, during butter melting and storage overnight, adding in ghee boiler before clarification or at final stage of clarification.

iv) Addition of dahi to butter before heating.

Similarly cooked flavour may be created or simulated in dairy ghee. Cooked flavour is the result of intense heat treatment in the presence of solid-not –fat component and for longer period of time. It is for this reason ghee produced from cream is rich in cooked flavour. Cooked flavour could be simulated by clarifying butter at temperatures above 115°C-120°C for 10 minutes and higher temperatuires without holding period. This could also be achieved by clarifying milk fat at different temperature and time and blending in different proportions.

Market Quality of Ghee

Consumer judge the quality of ghee based on its inherent flavour, colour and appearance. Ghee should have characteristic pleasant, nutty and slightly cooked rich aroma. Ghee flavour is best described as lack of blandness, sweet rather than acid. Golden yellow to light yellow colour of ghee is appreciated largely. Granular appearance of the product fetches more acceptance as it is an important quality criterion as well as purity parameter of ghee.

Apart from above sensory characteristics, its chemical and other physical parameters are evaluated to assess the quality of ghee. These physico-chemical parameters are also used as an indicator to detect any adulteration in ghee.

Refractive Index (RI) **:** It is defined as the ratio of the velocity of light in vacuum to the velocity of light in the sample medium. More generally, it is expressed as the ratio between the sine of the angle of incidence to the sine of the angle of refraction when a ray of light of a definite wave length passes from air into the fat. The reading is normally made at 40°C using Abbe-refractometer and its values normally range from 1.4157 to 1.4566. The RI of ghee is influenced by both the molecular weight and the degree of saturation of the constituent fatty acids. It could be used as an indicator of adulteration as its value for ghee is low in comparison to the other fats and oils.

Iodine Number **:** It is defined as number of grams of iodine absorbed by 100 g of fat under specified conditions. It measures degree of unsaturation in ghee. Compare to other fats and oils it is low for ghee. It is estimated using Wig's method. One molecule of halogen compound is absorbed by each unsaturated linkage and the absorption is expressed as the equivalent number of grams of iodine absorbed by 100 g of fat. Its value for milk fat is within the range of 26 to 35.

Reichert-Meissl Number (RM Number) **:** It is defined as the number of ml of N/10 sodium hydroxide required to neutralize the steam volatile water soluble fatty acids distilled from 5g of ghee under precise conditions specified in the method. It is primarily a measure of butyric acid and caproic acid. Its value for milk fat ranges from 17 to 35 and comparatively this value is higher than that of all other fats and oils, as milk fat contains more of these fatty acids than any other fats and oils.

Polenske Number **:** It is defined as number of ml of N/10 sodium hydroxide required to neutralize the steam volatile water insoluble fatty acids distilled from 5 g of fat under precise conditions specified in the method. Caprylic acid, capric acid which are steam volatile but largely insoluble in water are responsible for Polenske number and its value for ghee ranges from 12 to 24.

Saponification Number **:** It is defined as the number of milligrams of potassium required to saponify one gram of fat. Its value ranges from 210 to 233 and more often falls in the range of 225 to 230. It represents the average molecular weight of the fatty acid present in milk fat. It is more useful in detecting the presence of minerals oils such as liquid paraffin in ghee as they are not acted upon by alkali therefore the ghee sample containing such oils doesn't form a homogeneous solution on saponification.

Melting Point **:** Melting point for milk fat ranges from 30°C to 41°C as reported in literature. If there is an wider range then product should be further analyzed for confirmation of adulterants.

Factors Influencing the Market Quality of Ghee

Raw-materials (milk, dahi, cream or butter) used for ghee making: Milk used should be clean, fresh and strained. Butter made from ripened cream tends to improve the flavour score for ghee.

Type of feed **:** It is the main factor affecting variation in fatty acid composition of milk fat. The roughages present in the feed mainly consist of cellulose, which contribute to the formation of fatty acids of 4 to 16 carbon chain length. The lipid content of the feed contributes to the formation of long chain fatty acids of C_{16} and above. Animals fed with cotton seed meal show higher amount of C_{10} and C_{12} fatty acids.

Season **:** Another major factor which affects the texture of ghee. The granulation is more in winter and in monsoon season due to changes in the fatty acid profile. Also, ghee prepared in winter has higher acidity, melting point and grain size where as that of summer has the high saponification value.

Method of preparation **:** Flavour compounds of ghee vary according to its method of preparation (see flavour of ghee), for example ghee produced by *desi* method have more volatile carbonyl compounds than other methods. It was reported that ripening of cream reduces the keeping quality of ghee (Singh *et al.,* 1979). Ghee produced from Direct Cream method is more stable than that produced by the Creamery Butter method. This is because of longer duration of heat treatment in Direct Cream method that causes release of more number of phospholipids (acts as antioxidants).

Temperature of clarification : The temperature of clarification does have an influence on the quantity of carbonyl compounds and lactones formation. Higher temperature or longer period of heating at a particular temperature has been shown to higher stability during storage due to greater release of phospholipids.

Grading of Ghee "AGMARK Standards"

AGMARK is a certification mark of Government of India to ensure the purity and quality of Agricultural and allied products in India. The word 'AGMARK' is a derivative of "Agricultural Marketing". The Agricultural Produce (Grading & Marking) Act, 1936 empowers the Central Government to prescribe the quality standards, known as 'AGMARK' standards with terms and conditions to 'AGMARK' seal on individual packs. The Act empowers the Directorate of Marketing and Inspection to provide grade designation indicating the quality of the produce, to specify the manner in which the article could be packed, sealed and marked and to authorize a person or a body of persons to use the grade designation marks under prescribed condition. According to the law it is not compulsory for every trader and manufacturer, to get this AGMARK certification, therefore AGMARK is only a voluntary scheme of the Government.

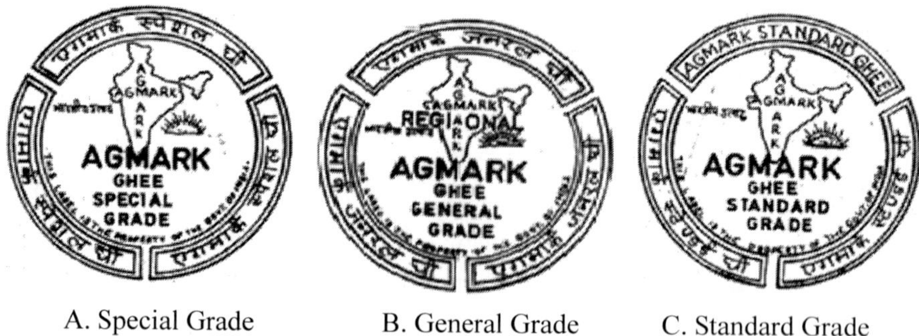

A. Special Grade B. General Grade C. Standard Grade

Fig. 6.13: AGMARK grade designations for ghee

Objectives of AGMARK

i. To assure the consumer and producer of pre-tested quality and purity

ii. To enable manufacturers of high grade product to obtain better returns

iii. To develop an orderly marketing of the commodities by eliminating malpractices when transferring from producer to consumer.

AGMARK Ghee Specifications

Grade designation marks for ghee: The grade designation mark shall consist of a label specifying the name of the commodity, grade designation and bearing a design consisting of an outline map of India with the word "AGMARK" and the figure of rising sun with the words produce of India and resembling the design as shown in figure 6.13. The letter and circular border colour should be red, green and chocolate for special, general and standard grade respectively. The labels shall be printed on the watermark paper of the Government of India and shall have a micro tint back ground bearing the words "Government of India" in olive green color. Each label shall have printed thereon a serial number along with a letter or letters denoting the series, e.g. A054987. Each label shall have printed thereon the approximate weight content of the package on which it is affixed.

Table 6.7: AGMARK standards of ghee

Parameters	Special Grade	General Grade	Standard Grade
Baudouin Test	Negative	Negative	Negative
BR reading at 40^{0}C	40.0– 43.0	40.0– 43.0	40.0– 43.0
Reichert Meissl value	Not less than 28.0	Not less than 28.0	Not less than 28.0
Polenske value	1.0 – 2.0	1.0 – 2.0	1.0 – 2.0
Moisture content (%)	Not more than 0.3	Not more than 0.3	Not more than 0.3
FFA (as % oleic acid)	Not more than 1.4	Not more than 2.5	Not more than 3.0

For cotton tracts areas such as part of Saurashtra and Madya Pradesh standards given table 6.8 are applicable.

Table 6.8: AGMARK standards for ghee produced in cotton tract areas

Parameters	Special Grade	
	Winter	Summer
Baudouin Test	Negative	Negative
BR reading at 40^{0}C	41.5 – 43.0	42.5 – 45.0
Reichert Meissl value	Not less than 23.0	Not less than 21.0[#]
Polenske value	0.5– 1.2	0.5 – 1.0
Moisture content (%)	Not more than 0.3%	Not more than 0.3%
FFA (as % oleic acid)	Not more than 1.4	Not more than 2.5

General and Standard grade have Percentage of Free Fatty Acids (as Oleic acid) shall not exceed 2.5 and 3.0 respectively.

Requirements of High Grade Ghee

Three main attributes of ghee are taste and aroma (flavour), granularity (texture) and colour. Superior quality ghee is the one which have following characteristics.

1. ***Flavour**:* Natural sweet and pleasant odour, an agreeable taste and it should be free from rancidity and any other objectionable falvour. A pleasant, nutty, slightly cooked aroma is appreciable in the product.
2. ***Texture**:* A large uniform grain with very little liquid fat is desirable, greasy texture is objectionable. Upon melting ghee should be clear, transparent and free from sediment and foreign colouring matter.
3. ***Colour**:* The colour should be uniform throughout, cow milk ghee should be bright yellow in colour and buffalo milk ghee should be white with or without a yellow or greenish tint.

Score card of Ghee

Ghee can be evaluated using the descriptive score card given in (Table 6.9).

Table 6.9: Score card of ghee

Characteristics	Maximum score
Colour	10
Flavour	50
Texture	30
Freedom from suspension	5
Package	5

Deductions of marks is based on degree of defects.

Characteristics	Defect	Degree of defects		
		Suspicion	Slight	Pronounced
Colour and appearance (10)	Brown	1	5	5
Colour and appearance (10)	Brown	1	5	5
Flavour (50)	Curdy	1	3	15
	Burnt	3	5	15
	Rancid	3	5	15
	Oxidized	1	3	15
	Smoky	1	3	10
Texture (30)	Greasy	3	5	15
	Hard	3	5	15
Suspended impurities (10)	Ghee residue	1	3	5

Note: Values in parenthesis indicates maximum score for sensory attribute

Defects of Ghee

Possible defects in ghee are discussed below with their causes and prevention. Defects are categorized according to the sensory characteristics such as flavor related, texture related and colour and appearance related.

1. Colour and appearance defects

a. ***Brown colour*** : This defect is due to the excessively high temperature of clarification. Optimum clarification temperature should be maintained during preparation of ghee.

b. ***Sediment*** : This defect is due to incorrect straining of ghee. Strainer should be able to retain all the sediment. Also, clarifier used for separating residue content should be place on smooth surface and should be efficient to separate ghee residue to the maximum extent.

2. Flavour defects

a. ***Smoky flavour*** : This defect is to the use of wood/cow dung cake as heating medium for boiling of milk/cream/butter that produces smoky fire.

b. ***Overcooked or bunt flavour*** : Excessively high temperature (beyond 118°C) of clarification causes this defect. This results in sudden rise in temperature and burning of curd causing burnt flavour. Therefore one has to be careful during final stage of ghee preparation.

c. ***Undercooked flavour*** : Excessively low temperature (80-100°C) of clarification causes this defect. Here the curd is not properly heated to release the flavoring compounds; such ghee also contains high moisture resulting in lower shelf life. Therefore optimum clarification temperature needs to be maintained.

d. ***Rancid flavour*** : This is due to hydrolysis of fat by lipase action in milk/cream /*dahi*/butter/ghee. Some of the heat resistant lipase enzymes released form psychrotrophes are difficult to destroy during heating. Therefore longer storage of milk or cream at refrigerated temperature before pasteurization should be avoided. Further, minimum moisture content in ghee prolongs the initiation of rancid flavour.

e. ***Oxidized/oily/metallic flavour*** : Presence of oxygen induces the oxidative changes in ghee. Therefore, filling ghee up to the brim helps to reduce the oxygen content in the pack. Also, flushing with nitrogen gas prevents the oxidative changes in ghee during storage. Contact with metals such as iron and copper catalyses the oxidative changes as well as imparts metallic flavour to ghee. Apart from this, direct exposure to sunlight also causes the oxidative changes in ghee. Also, another indirect factor responsible for oxidative changes is storage temperature, storage at higher temperature (>21°C) speed up the oxidative changes in ghee.

3. Texture defects

a. ***Greasy texture*** : After ghee preparation, if it is subjected to repeated heating and cooling treatments than greasy texture defect occur. Also, rapid cooling after clarification can also cause this defect. Therefore, after ghee is prepared, it is allowed to cool naturally before filtration and gradually cooled granulation.

Adulterants in Ghee

Milk fat is expensive among all the edible fats and oils. People therefore explore several ways to adulterate milk fat with cheaper source of fats/oils to make profits illegally. Adulteration of ghee in India is more prevalent especially in unorganized sector. Major adulterants of ghee are as follows:

i. Vanaspati (Hydrogenated vegetable oil). Because of close resemblance in its texture it is most commonly used as an adulterant to ghee.
ii. Refined (de-odourized) vegetable oil.
iii. Animal body fat.

Government has made it compulsory that all vanaspati must contain a maximum of 5% of sesame oil which can be identified in ghee by a simple colour test (known as Baudouin test). By means of this adulteration of ghee with vanaspati to an extent of 3% can be detected.

Use of Substandard Milk for Ghee Production

India, being a tropical country, ambient temperatures touches the mark of 40°C in summer in many places. Raw milk collection from rural area being carried out at ambient temperature causes acidity of milk to increase rapidly and results in souring of milk. This milk cannot withstand further thermal processing.

Therefore, there is a need to utilize this milk for products preparation without compromising the quality. So, in commercial dairy plants such milk is diverted and collected separately based on platform tests (COB, sensory etc.). This soured milk is collected in balance tank and circulated for 30 minutes using high speed pump. This provides effect similar to churning and causes the breakdown of fat globule membrane hence releases the free fat. Then fat is allowed to separate by gravity. Then this cream is used for ghee production either directly or collected over-a-period of time and neutralized to produce butter out of it, resultant butter could be used for ghee making. Ghee manufactured from neutralized milk or cream may differ from that prepared from fresh milk. Ghee made from sour milk has high liquid portion and comparatively dull colour.

Ghee As a Medicine

Milk fat contributes unique characteristics to the appearance, texture, flavour and satiability of dairy foods. It is an excellent source of energy, fat soluble vitamins and other potential health promoting components that perform various physiological functions in the body. Ghee has been ascribed a very important place as a medicine in Indian medicine or Ayurvedic treatmen*a*. As early as 1500 BC ghee was produced and known as *Ghritam, Sarpish, Havish* and *Ajya*. Rigveda contains numerous references on ghee showing its importance in Indian diet. The medicinal properties of ghee have been elucidated in a therapy called "Govaidak" that uses medicated ghee for treatment of several diseases. *Ayurveda* has identified ghee as a "*Madhura Rasa*" that can be used from birth. Ghee and honey mixture is given to new born babies in some part of India. Ghee is observed to improve the growth rate and digestibility. It also improves digestibility of other foods components. It has been reported that when cow ghee was added in diet, it increases digestibility of protein by 36% and biological value by 62%. The peak absorption of ghee occurs rapidly than other vegetable fats. The health benefits of ghee can be fundamentally categorized as (1) those that are obtained from consuming ghee as a food and (2) those that are obtained by using ghee as a medicine. *Ayurveda* text have described eight mammalian ghee namely – cow, buffalo, goat, sheep, camel, elephant, mare and human milk fat ghee to be useful for medication purposes. However, for majority of medicinal usage cow ghee is mostly preferred. The medicinal characteristic of different types of ghee obtained from different sources are described below:

(a) Cow milk ghee is said to be good for eyes and increases virility, appetite, radiance and intelligence capabilities.

(b) Buffalo milk ghee is heavy on digestion and proves remedial in haemolysis. Goat ghee is light in digestion, appetizing, eye invigorating and strength increasing.

(c) Eve milk ghee is light in digestion and beneficial in rigour and phthisis.

(d) Camel milk ghee is appetizing, anti toxic and pungent in digestion. It is beneficial in treatment of cutaneous infection, abdominal glands, worms, oedema and ascites.

(e) Mare milk ghee is light in digestion, anueretic and astringent in taste.

(f) Elephant milk ghee is helpful in treatment of worms, poisoning and cutaneous infection.

(g) Human milk ghee is light in digestion, anti toxic, appetizing and good for eye diseases.

The major difference lies in method of production that may change the levels of micronutrients in ghee. Some prefer production of ghee from fresh milk while some prefer the fermentation process. Fermentation may lead to changes in the activity of particular component in food system and that may lead to change in health benefits of ghee prepared by different methods. The medicinal properties of ghee made from un-fermented (fresh milk) and fermented milk has been differentiated by *Ayurveda*. It says that ghee made from fresh milk is cool and beneficial for eye diseases. It eliminates blood impurities and is beneficial for diarrhea. While fermented milk ghee is good as an appetizer, provides strength and virility, eliminates fevers and beneficial for eyes. Old ghee is considered immensely superior for external usage. It has been used for treatment of various skin diseases. Various classes of old/stored ghee, depending on storage period are:

i) *Puran ghee* – That is proximate one year old and is effective in treatment of coma, ear and eye diseases and healing of wounds

ii) *Kumbha ghee* – That is proximately 11-100 years old. This ghee is used for treatment of cough, epileptic fits, skin problems and fever.

iii) *Maha ghee* – That is stored for more than 100 years. This ghee is generally used for wound healing and massage.

Preparation of Medicated Ghee

The *Ayurveda* pharmacopoeia described about 50-60 types of medicated ghee and their usage in treatment of various diseases. Medicated ghee is generally prepared with fortification of selected herbs in order to extract fat soluble therapeutic components from herbs. Depending upon the type of herb used and the form in which it is used (liquid, paste, powder) different treatment are given during manufacture of medicated ghee of different types. However, the generalized method, described in a classic *Ayurveda* text "*Sharangdhar samhita*", is to mix 4 parts of ghee and 1 part of herb in 16 parts of water. The mixture is brought to boiling till all water is evaporated. The resultant product is then filtered/clarified and allowed to cool at room temperature. The cooled ghee is then filled in required containers and stored.

Usage

Medicated ghee is used both in external and internal applications. Generally fresh medicated ghee is used for external purposes like massage and eye treatment, in the form of paste. The internal applications involves cleaning of upper gut, treatment of G.I. disorders, nasal administration through oral ingestion.

Table 6.10: Medicated ghee in ayurvedic treatment

Medicated ghee type (ghirt)	Treatment for	Medicated ghee type (ghirt)	Treatment for
Arjuna ghirt	Heart disease	*Amruta* ghirt	Leprosy
Amrutparsh ghirt	Anti aging	*Ashwagandha* ghirt	GI disorders
Kushadhya ghirt	Stones	*Kantakari* ghirt	Cough
Changeri ghirt	Immunopotentiation	*Chitrak* ghirt	Spleen/Liver
Dadimadi ghirt	Anemia	*Dhanvantar* ghirt	Diabetes
Patoladhya ghirt	Eyes	*Panchgavya* ghirt	Hysteria
Shatavari ghirt	Ulcer	*Manha shiladi* ghirt	Asthama
Maha badrick ghirt	Leucodarma	*Som* ghirt	Infertility
Chagladhya ghirt	Tuberclosis	*Varunadi* ghirt	Piles
Kumar kalyan ghirt	Child disorders	*Kalyan* ghirt	Madness

Source : Ayurvedic Pharmacopoeia (1963)

Butter Oil

Conversion of butter or cream into butter oil is a means to preserve excess fat, produced/obtained during peak milk production periods. The terms anhydrous milk fat, dehydrated butter fat and dry butter fat are used synonymously with butter oil.Butter oil refers to the fat concentrate obtained mainly from butter or cream by the removal of practically all the water and solid not fat content. Butter oil lacks the flavour of Indian ghee.

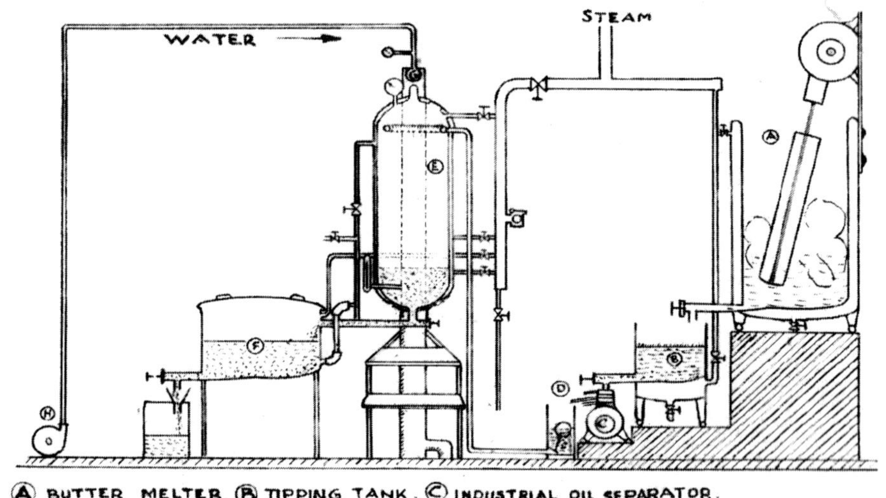

Fig. 6.14: Butter oil plant

Table 6.11: Chemical Composition of Butter oil

Constituents	Percentage
Moisture	0.1-0.2
Milk fat	99.5-99.8
Free acid (%oleic)	0.2-0.5
Peroxide value	0.0-0.1

FSSAI Definition

Butter-oil, anhydrous milk fat / anhydrous butter-oil means the fatty products derived exclusively from milk and / or products obtained from milk by means of process which results in almost total removal of water and solid-not fat contents. It shall have pleasant taste and flavour free from off-odour and rancidity. It shall be free from vegetable oil/ fat, animal body fat, mineral oil, added flavour and any other substance foreign to milk. It may contain food additives permitted in these regulation including in appendix A. (permitted anti-oxidants not exceeding 0.02 % by weight except gallate which shall not exceed 0.01 per cent by weight). It shall confirm to the microbiological requirements prescribed in appendix B.

It shall confirm to following requirements:-

Requirements	Milk fat / Butter-oil	Anhydrous milk fat
BR reading (at 40 C)	40 - 44	40 - 44
Moisture (%)	Not more than 0.40	Not more than 0.10
Milk fat (%)	Not less than 99.60	Not less than 99.80
RM Value	Not less than 24	Not less than 24
FFA (% Oleic acid)	Not more than 0.40	Not more than 0.30
Peroxide value (m.eq. oxygen/kg fat)	Not more than 0.60	Not more than 0.30
Boudouin test	Negative	Negative

Product Description

Looks similar to ghee, pale yellow liquid, majorly constitute of milk fat. Alternatively it can be called as anhydrous milk fat (AMF). According to FAO/ WHO AMF should have min 99.8% fat.

Methods of Preparation

Butter oil may be prepared from cream or butter.

1. Industrial production of butteroil from cream (de-emulsification process)

Raw cream of 35-40% fat content is pasteurized through plat heat exchanger or tubular heat exchanger. Then it passes through cream concentrator (essentially cream separator) to achieve a fat percent level of around 75-78%. Here we can store the cream as intermediary storage. Cream is then fed to homogenizer for phase inversion (it breaks the fat globule membrane to release the fat). After phase inversion product again pass through centrifugal concentrator where the cream fat level is rise to 99.5%. Heating will be done at 95 to 98°C in a plate heat exchanger. Reduce the moisture content of the product to 0.1% in vacuum chamber followed cooling to ambient temperature through PHE.

Butter is transferred to butter melting vat, where it is heated to 60°C to 80°C.Transferred to holding tank, where it is hold for 20-30 min to facilitate protein aggregation. Then butter melt is transferred to centrifugal concentrator, where light phase is concentrated to 99.5% fat. Concentrated light phase is then pumped through plate heat exchanger (PHE) where it is heated to 90-95°C. Then to vacuum chamber for final moisture adjustment then back to PHE for cooling to 35-40°C before packing.

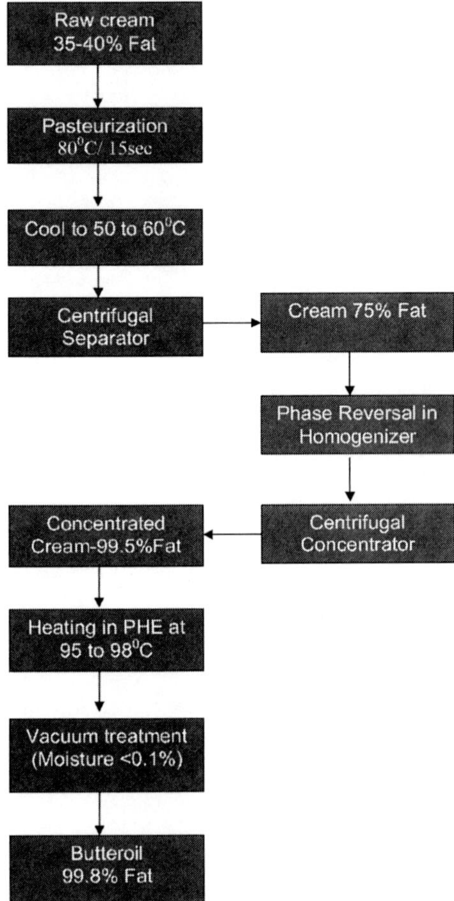

Fig. 6.15: Industrial production of butteroil from cream

The method of manufacture consists of slowly heating the butter till it melts then the temperature is gradually raised to 108°-110° C. When all the moisture has evaporated, the residual butter fat is drained from the curd and filtered. Alternatively, the butter after melting is left undisturbed to stratitify into serum, fat and serum layers. The fat layer is then drawn and cooled. Both these methods are batch process where the recovery is low and are only suitable for samll scale manufacture of butteroil.

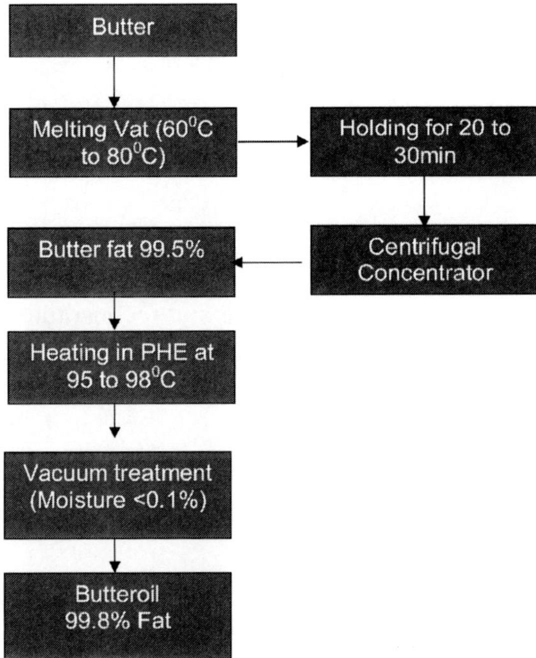

Fig. 6.16: Industrial production of butteroil from butter

The centrifugal separation and vacuum drying method is continuous and yields high quality product. The typical method is melting of butter in a double jacketed vat fitted with variable speed agitator. The melted butter is allowed to enter the oil separator gradually so that the melt separates into oil and serum. The oil passes through the balance tank into the vacuum pan where it is hydrated at 56°-63° under vacuum (57-62 Cm mercury). At the end of the operation the butter oil is allowed to flow by gravity into receiving kettle for subsequent cooling (13-18°C), packaging and storage at room temperature.

Packaging and Storage

Butteroil is filled in containers of various sizes. Filling should be done up to the brim in the container in such a manner as to exclude maximum oxygen. For households and restaurants containers of 1 kg to 20 kg are available. For industrial uses drums of minimum 180kg are also available. An inert gas, nitrogen, is used for packing to prevent oxidation. Care should be taken to exclude oxygen when packing butter oil in the containers. To enhance shelf life anti oxidants like Ethyl gallate (0.005-0.01%) and hydroquinine (0.01-0.10%) etc may be added before packaging depending upon health regulations and based on use of permitted antioxidants only. Alternatively the product is packed under 500 mm vacuum prior to sealing.

Butteroil can be stored at ambient temperature since it contains very low amount of moisture, expected shelf life of product at this storage temperature is about one year.

Uses of Butteroil

It is used in the production of recombined and reconstituted milk, cream and butter. It can also be used in the manufacture of ice cream and in the confectionery industry as a source of fat. Butteroil is also utilized in the production of various types of fat spreads. It can be used for the manufacture of toffee and chocolate and as a cooking fat. Coversion of cream and butter to butteroil is a convenient method of preservation of milk fat where refrigerated storage is not available.

Suggested Readings

Abichandani, H, Sarma, S.C. and Bector, B.S., (1991). Continuous ghee manufacture. An engineering solution. Ind food industry,10(4):35-37.

Abichandani, H., Bector, B.S. and Sarma, S.C. (1995). Continuous ghee making system-design, operation and performance. Ind. J Dairy Sci., 48: 646.

Acharya, K.T. (1997). Ghee, vanaspati and special fats in India. In: Lipid Technology and applications. Ed.F.D.Gunstone and F.B. Padley. Marcel Deckker Inc., New York. Pp.369-90.

Arumughan, C. and Narayanan, K.M. (1979). Grain formation in ghee. J. Food Sci. Technology, 16:242-247.

Banerjee, A.K. (1997). Processes for commercial production. In: Dairy India, 5th Edn., pp. 387.

Bector, B.S., Abichandani, H. and Sarma, S.C. (1996). Shelf life of ghee manufactured in continuous ghee making system. Ind. J Dairy Sci., 49: 398

Chakraborty, B.K. (1980). Industrial ghee production- Trends and innovations. Paper presented at IDA Ghee Conference. Sept.-12-13.

Dairy Handbook. Alfa Laval AB, Dairy and Food Engineering Division S-22103 Lund, Sweden.

Dave,G.K.; Dave, R.H. and Dave, N.G. (1991). Panchakarma Kalpana. Saraswati Pustak Bhandar, Ahmedabad, India.

Edger Spreer (1998) Milk and Dairy Product Technology. Marcel Dekker Inc. New York.

Galhotra, K.K. and Wadhwa, B.K. (1993). Chemistry of ghee residue, its significance and utilization-A review. Ind. J. Dy. Sci.,46:142.

Ganguli, N.C. and Jain, M.K. (1973). Ghee: its chemistry, processing and Technology. J. Dairy Sci., 56:19-25.

Gorden, M. (1991). Monograph on utilization of milk fat. IDF Bulletin No. 260.

Hamilton, R.J. and Rossel, J.B. (1986). Analysis of oils and fats. Elsevier Applied Science Publishers Ltd., London.

More GR (1987). Progress of the project, NDRI Annual Report pp 89-90.

Mortensen, B.K. (1983). Physical properties and modification of milk fat. In: Developments in dairy chemistry. Vol.II. ed.P.A.Fox. Applied science publication.

Pandya,T.N.(1996). *Ghrit.* Ayu Research Jr.,17(9):1-4.

Punjrath J.S. (1974). New developments in ghee making. Indian Dairyman,26: 275.

Punjrath, J.S., Kumar, R. and Bandyopadhyay, P. (1997). Tapping the potential of traditional dairy foods. In Souvenir: 28th Dairy Industry Conference, Bangalore April 27-29.

Rajorhia, G.S. (1993). Ghee. Encyclopaedia of Food Science, Food Technology and Food Nutrition, Academic Press, London, pp 2186.

Richard Bolten, E.R. (1999). Oils, fat and fatty foods. Biotech Books Publisher, Delhi.

Serunjogi, M.L., Abramsen, R.K. and Narvhus, J. (1998). Current knowledge of ghee and related products-A review. International Dairy J., 8(8):677-88.

Wadhwa, B.K. (1995). Chemistry of ghee and ghee residue. Indian Dairyman, 47:32.

Wadhwa, B.K. and Bindal, M.P. (1995). Ghee residue : a promise for stimulating flavours in vanaspati and butteroil. Indian J.Dairy Sci., 48:469.

Wadhwa, B.K. and Jain M.K. (1990). Chemistry of ghee flavor – a review. Indian J. Dairy Sci., 48:601.

Yadav, J.S. and Srinivasan, R.A. (1992). Advances in ghee flavor research. Indian J.Dairy Sci.,45:338.

Zaveri, K. (2000). Hridayrog. Bansali Trust, Surat, India.

7

Nutritional Aspect of Milk Fat

Introduction

In the recent past there has been a great deal of questioning regarding role of milk fat in cholesterol metabolism and other body functions. The enormous wave against cholesterol containing foods has damaged the image and market growth of fat rich dairy products. This trend is due to presence of saturated fats and cholesterol that are known to increase the incidence of coronary heart diseases one of the common cause of heart attack. The educated and urban society is more health conscious about the presence of cholesterol in their diets. This has led to the greater demand of cholesterol free foods. Ghee being a saturated fat and containing little amount of cholesterol, is suspected to contribute towards coronary heart diseases. However, critically surveyed scientific literature indicates that there is no evidence of any association of milk fat with increased risk of coronary heart diseases. Age old and proven Ayurvedic system of medicine has proved the usage of ghee to induce several beneficial effects on human health and used extensively for therapeutic purpose like in treatment of skin allergy, respiratory diseases, curative for ulcers and eye diseases. This suggest that ghee is a valuable form of dietary fat.

Dietary fat should provide 15% of total energy of which 20% should come from essential fatty acids. A minimum visible fat requirement should be 20g per person per day. The type and composition of dietary fat is important for human health. Lipid the most important constituent of milk, play a very significant role in human nutrition. They are the rich source of fat soluble vitamins (ADEK) and essential fatty acids, apart from having pleasant sensory attributes. It contains number of components like- sphingomyleine, beta-carotene and conjugated linoleic acids (CLA) which shows anti-carcinogenic activity. Milk fat is composed of tri-glyceride (96-99%), di-glycerides (0.3-1.0%), phospholipids (0.1-0.3%), cholesterol (0.2-.04%) and free fatty acids (0.1-0.4%). The major fatty acid in milk fat is palmetic (24-28%), oleic (23-28%), myristic (13-14%) and stearic (11-12%). It is good source of vitamin A (900-1200IU/100g) of which carotene contributes to 30% in cow milk fat. It also contains vitamin D (20-60IU/100g) and vitamin E 92.6-3.5mg/100g). Milk fat even being consisting of short chain fatty acids, is easily digested because of its fatty acid composition and state of dispersion. Milk fat globules can be absorbed without preceeding enzymic hydrolysis. Milk fat is a valuable dietary constituent with a therapeutic potential in diseases of stomach. liver, intestine, kidney and gall bladder. Short chain fatty acids also promote growth of major probiotic bacteria, Bifidus bacteria, in the intestine. Milk fat also contains high content of medium chain fatty acids which are easily and directly absorbed by the blood of portal vein into the system. The degree of digestibility of milk fat is 99%. The digestibility is effected by the position of fatty acid on the triglyceride molecule. Short chain fatty acids are mainly found at the outer position and are first attacked by lipase enzyme producing 1,2 diglyceride followed by 2 monoglyceride. Milk fat is best absorbed in the form of monoglycerides and fatty acids. Short chain fatty acids with 4-12 carbon atoms are reported to have anti-microbial activity that can inhibit growth of gram negative organisms. Milk fat also contains unique fatty acids and other potential therapeutic micro-nutrients like Conjugated linoleic acids (CLA), vaccinic acid and butyric acids that are beneficial for human health in providing protection against colon cancer by associating with dawn regulation or inactivation of cancer genes. Conjugated linoleic acids (CLAs) are a group of naturally occurring isomers of linoleic acid containing a conjugated double bond system. It is formed in the rumen as intermediate product in digestion of dietary fats. Different CLA isomers are present in milk and milk products from ruminant animals and are of great interest with respect to their anti-carcinogenic effect. In fact, CLA is the only fatty acid that has clearly been shown to reduce cancer in experimental animals as well as in humans.. a number of studies indicate that CLA inhibits human malignant melanoma and colorectal, breast, lung and ovarian cancer cell lines. Besides the anti-carcinogenic effects of CLA isomers, they have also been reported to exhibit several biological activities such as reduction in atherosclerosis, increase in bone mass and muscle mass. They have also shown immuno-modulating properties. CLA isomers that originate from linoleic acids in the rumen are the major contributors to CLA in dairy products. Milk and milk products are the richest source of CLA.

CLA is an potential anti- mutagenic substance and is most abundantly present in ghee. Consumption of ghee increases CLA content in mammary tissues several folds. The CL:A content of dairy products varies from 0.6-30mg/g fat. It is not only powerful anti-carcinogen, it also has anti-atherogenic, immuno-modulating and growth promoting properties. Dietary CLA at 1% level has been shown to inhibit mammary tumors. CLA may be beneficial in preventing some diseases by modulating lipid metabolism and immune functions thus causing delay or even inhibiting on set of diseases like cancer, diabetic and atheroclerosis. The cis-trans isomer of linoleic acid in milk fat has been identified as an inhibitor of cancerous growth in colon and mammary glands. Milk has been shown to have anti-cholesteromic affect in human. Both decreased biosynthesis and increased cholesterol break down to bile acid in liver are the likely reasons for hypo-cholestromic affect of milk fat. The presence of Orotic acid and other neucleotides associated with proteose-peptone fraction of milk are believed to have cholesterol lowering properties.

Inclusion of vegetable oils with the purpose of reducing serum cholesterol levels have resulted in increased number of non-cardiovascular deaths especially cancer. In fact excess consumption of poly-unsaturaed faty acid rich vegetable oils have been suggested to actually promote atherogenesis owing to its nature to oxidative modification. Lowering of serum cholesterol by PUFA rich vegetable oils is attributed to re distribution of cholesterol in body tissues. An increased excretion of cholesterol in the form of bile acids may accelerate formation of gall stones and also leads to increased colonization of intestine with bile degrading bacteria. Excessive intake of PUFA increases vitamin E requirement because of its oxidative products that causes alteration in membrane of blood carpocels

Dietary Value

Milk fat is relatively high in short chain and medium chain fatty acids which have been reported to have antimicrobial activity. These fatty acids have fungicidal and bactericidal effect against certain acid resistant bacteria and moulds. The short chain fatty acids in milk fat also promote growth of *Lactobacillus bifidum* in intestine. The cis-trans isomer of linoleic acid, identified in milk, appears to be an inhibitor of cancerous growth in colon and mammary gland. The important role of milk fat in particular is to enhance the food value. Milk fat is a good source of fat soluble vitamins like Vitamin A (1000-2000 IU/100 g), Vitamin D (20-60 IU/100 g) and Vitamin E (2.6-3.5 mg/100g).

Digestability

Milk fat is easily digestable as compared to other fats and oils. The high content of short and medium chain fatty acids in milk fat are more easily absorbed than long chain fatty acids. The degree of digestability of milkm fat is 99%. Short chain fatty acids are takenup directly by the portal vein in the form of free fatty acids. The milk fat globule particles can pass directly through lymphatic ducts and are able to penetrate intestinal epithelium at the tip of villi. Upon enzymatic breakdown of milk fat emulsion, the fine dispersion of mixture of diacylglycerol, monoacylglycerol and free fatty acids are absorbed by the mucosa. Because of the easy digestability and absorption of milk fat ,it puts little strain on the body.

Cholestrol Lowering Effect

Milk fat is often implicated with coronary heart diseases because of cholesterol content. However, the cholesterol content of milk fat is relatively low (1.9-2.8 mg/g). In contrast human body synthesizes higher amounts than absorbed. At any given time nearly 10-14g of cholesterol is present in blood. Several investigators have shown that milk has a hypocholesterolaemic effect in humans and experimental animals. Consumption of fat rich buffalo milk has been shown to lower the plasma cholesterol level in experimental animals. Many experiments involving human volunteers with daily intake of as much as two liters of milk have shown no rise in cholesterol level, contrary the cholesterol level was often reduced. Milk decreased the generation of NADPH a reductant required in cholesterol biosynthesis via pentose phosphate pathway of glucose oxidation. The decreased biosynthesis and increased breakdown of cholesterol have been reported to be the reason of hypocholesterolaemic effect of milk.

Suggested Readings

Aggarwal, R.A.K. and Kansal, V.K. (1991). Indian J. Med. Res., 94:147.

Aggarwal, R.A.K. and Kansal, V.K. (1991). Milchwiss., 46:355.

Aggarwal, R.A.K. and Kansal, V.K. (1992). Indian J. Med. Res., 96:55.

Aggarwal, R.A.K. and Kansal, V.K. (1993). Indian J. Dairy Sci., 46:104.

Gurr, M.L. (1981). J. Dairy Res., 48:519.

Hodgson, J.M. et. al. (1993). American J. Clin. Nutri., 58:228

Chawla, K. and Kansal, V.K. (1983). MIlchwiss., 38:1963

Kansal,V.K. and Chawla, K. (1984). Indian J. Nutri. Dietet., 21:54.

Srinivasan, S. and Kansal, V.K. (1988). Indian J. Dairy Sci.,41:469.

Srinivasan, S. and Kansal, V.K. (1986). Milchwiss., 41:136.

8

By–Products From Fat Rich Product Industry

Introduction

The economic choice of any process is the criterion for efficient utilization of the by-product that is produced along side of main product. During manufacture of major dairy products, the dairy industry also ends up in producing different by-products. Various by-products of dairy industry are skim milk, butter milk , whey and ghee residue. Dairy industry is particularly confronted with the problem of economic utilization of whey and ghee residue. The techno-economical problems associated with utilization of these by-products, is now receiving considerable attention. More efficient, cost effective and sophisticated technologies have opened up new vistas for manufacture of number of derived by-products. Further more the market for dairy by-products, as an ingredients in other consumer food products like snacks, ready meals and microwavable food products, has been growing. Indian dairy industry is trying to make advancement in this direction. This became possible after economic liberalisation and delicensing of dairy industry resulting in due attention to by-products processing. However, host of problems like type and quality of raw milk, lack of organized product manufacture, lack of adequate technology, high cost of importing new technologies, adequate infrastructure etc. are associated with production and utilization of by-products in India. Nevertheless, during recent years, number of manufacturing units with large automated and continuous manufacturing facilities for utilizing dairy by products have been set up in the country.

Skim Milk

It is a by-product obtained during manufacture of cream. It is rich in solid-not-fat content. It is a rich source of high quality milk proteins (casein and whey proteins), minerals (calcium, phosphorus, potassium, manganese, zinc, selenium, iron etc.) and water soluble vitamins (B-complex and vit. C). It is mainly utilized in standardization of fat content in dairy products to meet the legal standard. When in excess it is preserved in dried form (as skim milk powder) by removing moisture. It is therefore, not considered as by-product. However, it is regarded as by-product when it is utilized for manufacture of skim milk derived products such as casein and caseinates, co-precipitate or protein hydrolysate.

Casein

It is the major milk protein that makes up 80% of total milk protein. Casien exist in milk as a calcium caseinate-calcium phosphate complex. When pH is lowered by addition of acid to the skim milk, this complex is dissociated. Calcium is displaced from the casein molecule by hydronium ions and calcium phosphate complex is converted into soluble calcium ions and phosphate ions. At pH 5.3 the casein starts to precipitate and complete precipitation occurs at pH 4.6. Casein can be manufactured in both industrial and edible form depending upon its usage and demand. It can be manufactured either by addition of acid (mineral / food grade) or it can be removed from solution by enzymic coagulation process.

Casein may be typed according to the process used for precipitation - a) acid casein, b) rennet casein and c) coprecipitated casein. Casein precipitated by acid is usally includes the name of the acid in its description. Any of the acid (Hydrochloric, Sulphuric, Lactic acids) can be used for precipitation processes to produce both industrial and edible casein. The choice of method used for casein precipitation is largely governed by economics.

Manufacture of industrial casein does not warrant high quality skim milk. The skim milk is generally coagulated using any mineral acid that helps in reduction of milk pH to an iso-electric point of casein where it is precipitated out of solution. It is then collected , pressed to remove excess of moisture and finally grated, dried and grinded into fine particles and packed into poly-ethylene lined craft paper bags. Lactic casein is prepared by inoculating the skim milk with lactic acid producing cultures. A slow acid producing culture is preferred as it exhibit less proteolysis and increased protein yield. The process of coagulum formation generally takes about 14-16 hours. The coagulum is then cut into small pieces and cooked to creat firm curd for subsequent processing. Acid and heat help in synersis of whey. The use of mineral acids has the advantage of quick curd formation, shortening the coagulation time and also the operation can be made continuous. Hydrochloric acid is more superior coagulating agent which is used after 6-9 times dilution with portable water. A high grade casein having low ash content and high solubility is made by grain curd process. Here coagulation is attained at 35° C using diluted HCl to a pH value of 4.1 that produces granular curd which is easy to drain and wash. Casein in its industrial form (crude casein) has been associated with paper, textile, paint and leather industry since ages.

Manufacture of **edible casein** differs from non-edible casein by use of high heat treatment of skim milk, food grade chemicals and production under strict sanitary conditions. The process of making edible casein is efficient separation of fat from skim milk. Filtered and warm milk is separated in a hermetic separator to reduce fat to less than 0.05%. it is then pasteurized to achieve microbiological standard, before acidification with food grade acid, draining of whey, washing the resultant curd with pasteurized water. It is then pressed, grated and dried. Edible casein is an established dairy byproduct that is used as an ingredient in many dairy and food products. During recent two decades it has been used for fortification or admixture in other food products.

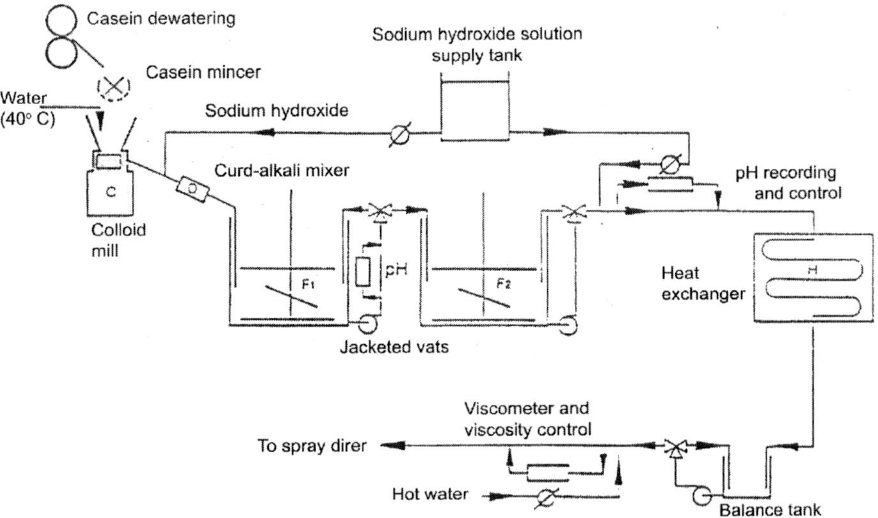

Fig. 8.1: Schematic for sodium caseinate manufacture

With advancement in technology and automation, continuous casein manufacturing units have been made possible for large production (14000-18000 l/hr). In continuous system provision exist for constant flow of milk and acid, accurate measurement of acid, controlling coagulation temperature and mixing for acid in milk to obtain complete coagulation and well structured curd. Washing of curd is done in three or five stages with holding time of 20-30 minutes. Pressing of curd is achieved through use of roller press or by decanters. There are several type of equipments for drying casein but widely used presently is the vibratory drier. The drier features fast revolving multi chambered rotor with serated surface. This grinds the curd to very fine particle thus increasing the surface area to the hot air that conveys the curd through the drier. Drying takes only few seconds and the product is similar to spray drier casein. Such plants reduces manufacturing cost, improves the value of milk protein and also elevate the status of casein for industrial and food usage.

Table 8.1: Standards for edible casein (National, International)

Constituents	ISI:1167–1965	FIL-IDF 45:1969	
		Standard grade	Extra grade
Moisture % max.	10	12	12
Total solids % max.			
Fat % max	1.5	2.25	1.7
Protein % max.	-	90	95
Acid insoluble ash % max.	0.1	-	-
Lactose % max.	-	1	0.2
Free acidity (ml of 0.1N NaOH) max.	5.6/10g	0.27/g	0.20/g
Copper max ppm	-	5	5
Iron max ppm	-	5	5
Lead max ppm	-	2.25	1.7
Bacterial count/g	50,000	100,000	30,000
Coliform count	10/g	Nil in 0.1g	Nil in 0.1g
Thermoduric/g	-	5,000	5,000
Yeast & mould/g	-	100	50

Casein and casein derivatives are widely used in bakery products for nutritional fortification of wheat flour and for flavour enhancement. Acid, rennet casein, sodium and calcium caseinate can be used in bread making to the level of 15-20% of wheat flour. Casein helps to improve dough making properties and texture of bakery products. Supplementation of wheat flour with casein improves the amino acid profile of resultant product and considerably increases the protein efficiency ratio (PER) value of the mixture. The important functional characteristic of casein product in bakery products is its water holding/binding capacity. Casein has the ability to bind twice their weight of water and thus producing an drying effect. It aid in blending by promoting emulsification and improving emulsion stability.

Caseinates are the soluble form of casein and prepared from freshly precipitated acid casein curd by reacting with diluted solution of alkali. Casein should have low calcium content (< 0.15%) to produce a caseinate solution with low viscosity and low lactose content (< 0.2%) on dry basis. There are many variants of caseinates that can be prepared and this depends on the type of alkali (sodium, potassium, calcium, magnesium hydroxides) used for solubilization purpose and the final usage. Sodium hydroxide is the most common alkali used. Irrespective of starting material used, the manufacture of sodium caseinate consists of formation of casein suspension, solubilization of casein using alkali (sodium hydroxide-2.5M solution) and drying of the prepared slurry having 20-30% total solids.

Table 8.2: Typical composition of caseinates

Constituents	Sodium caseinate	Calcium caseinate
Moisture (%)	3.8	3.8
Fat (%)	1.1	1.1
Protein % (Nx6.38)	91.4	91.2
Lactose (%)	0.1	0.1
Ash (%)	3.6	3.8
Sodium (%)	1.2-1.4	<0.1
Calcium (%)	0.1	1.3-1.6
Iron (mg/kg)	3 - 20	10 – 40
Lead (mg/kg)	<1.0	<1.0
pH	6.5 – 6.9	6.8 – 7.0

Source: Gupta 2008

Co-precipitate

During casein manufacture skim milk is precipitated by acidification. This results in recovery of only casein as a final product. The more nutritious whey proteins are lost in the whey. These nutritious whey proteins can be recovered by application of high heat treatment of skim milk before acidification. Precipitation of casein and whey proteins together from heated milk by acidification is termed as "Co-precipitate". The skim milk is heated to a temperature of 90°-95°C that helps to denature and induce complexation of whey proteins with casein, followed by precipitation of protein complex by acidification or combination of added calcium chloride (0.25%) and acidification (pH 4.6). Depending about usage of co-precipitate, the calcium content may vary and hence a range of co-precipitate s can be manufactured namely- Low (0.5-0.8%), Medium (1-2%) and high (2.5-3.0%) calcium co-precipitate. The level of calcium in the product is controlled by varying pH of precipitation, amount of calcium added and length of time for which the held at 90°-95°C. For low calcium co-precipitate calcium chloride is added at the rate of 0.03-0.04% and milk is held at 90°C for 12-15 minutes followed by acidification at pH 4.6. For medium calcium co-precipitate, calcium chloride is added at the rate of 0.06-0.08% with 10 minutes holding time of milk at 90°C and acidified at pH 5.4. High calcium co-precipitate is prepared by admixing 0.2% calcium chloride, holding milk at requisite temperature for 1-2 minutes followed by acidification. Precipitation at lower temperature and higher pH results in co-precipitate with poor solubility properties. However, a soluble lacto-protein may be manufactured by first adjusting skim milk pH to 7.5, heating in the range of 85°-90°C and holding for 15 to 20 minutes followed by cooling to 45°C and adjusting pH to 4.4-4.7 to precipitate the proteins. The curd is separated, washed, dispersed in water and dissolved at pH 6.7 before spray drying. The yield of co-precipitate is around 95-97%.

Table 8.3: Proximate composition of co-precipitates

Constituents	Co-precipitates		
	High calcium	Medium calcium	Low calcium
Moisture (%)	9.5	9.5	9.5
Fat (%)	0.6	0.7	0.9
Protein (%) (Nx6.38)	81.7	85.6	86.7
Protein (%) dry basis	90.3	94.5	95.8
Lactose (%)	0.5	0.5	0.5
Ash (%)	7.7	3.7	2.4
Calcium (%)	2.81	1.13	0.54
pH	7.1-7.2	6.6-7.1	6.6-7.2

Source: Southward 1985

Co-precipitates are used in variety of food products in small proportions to improve their functional and nutritive value. However, successful usage depends upon satisfactory functional properties of protein that are added in the food system so that body, texture and nutritive characteristics of finished product

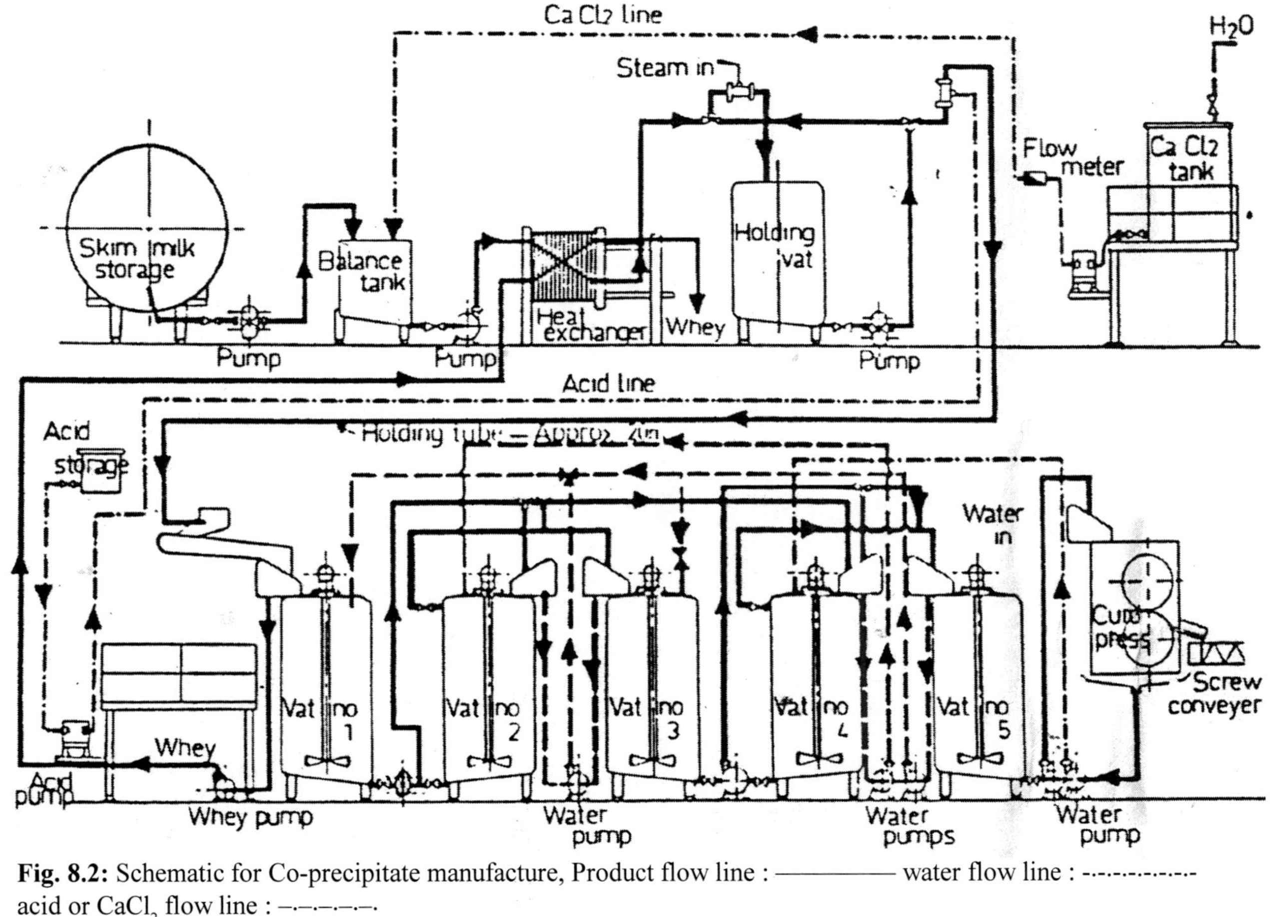

Fig. 8.2: Schematic for Co-precipitate manufacture, Product flow line : ———— water flow line : ------- acid or $CaCl_2$ flow line : —·—·—·

are not adversely affected. Also its usage must not change the flavor of finished product and remain acceptable to the consumers.

Protein Hydrolysate

Protein Hydrolysate are manufactured for utilization of protein rich food by product, waste and non conventional food proteins. Historically soy souce is the first protein hydrolysate. The flavor characteristic of protein hydrolysate is suggestive of meat flavor. However, protein hydrolysate manufactured from different sources of protein like fish, egg, soy, casein etc. have distinct flavor characteristics. Lighter and more delicate flavouredhydrolysates are derived from milk protein. Casein is an important substrate/raw material for the preparation of milk protein hydrolysate. Casein hydrolysate are manufactured by acid, alkali or enzymatic hydrolysis of casein.

Acid hydrolysis can be achieved by reacting casein or caseinate with hydrochloric acid or sulphuric acid for 4-18 hours at a temperature of 80°-100° C. Thereafter the contents are nutrilized to pH 6-7 by an alkali. The draw backs are complete or partial destruction of most of the amino acids. The process also hinders removal of residual acid and forms salts which becomes limiting factor for its usage in food and dietetic application. Use of alkali for hydrolysis is yet another process but is not an effective method as it causes destruction and recimisation of amino acids as well as destruction of functional groups of amino acid residues.

Enzymatic hydrolysis is the safest process for conversion of casein into high grade milk protein hydrolysate. Proteolytic enzymes obtained from various sources like plants (Papian, Ficin), animals (Pepsin, Trypsin, Rennin) and microbial (Pronase, Alcalase, Neutrase, Naturase) could be used for enzymic hydrolysis of milk protein. They have the ability to hydrolyse proteins And amino acids. The chain length of peptides formed is dependent on conditions applied and extent of hydrolysis, substrate and enzyme concentration and activity of the enzyme used. This process of casein hydrolysis results in high content of water soluble nitrogen and less salts. It causes no destruction or recemisation of amino acids and retains nutritive value of original protein. The choice of protease for protein hydrolysis depends on its specificity, pH optima, temperature(heat stability) and presence of acitivators or inhibitors. Selection of proper enzyme is important for obtaining desirable functionality in the resultant product. Enzymes with broad specificity that leads to extensive hydrolysis of proteins into low molecular weight peptides and amino acids is best suited for flavor purposes. Casein hydrolysate with improved flavor characteristics/ qualities can be manufactured by adding proteolytic enzyme in 10% casein solution (adjusted to pH 6-7) and reacted for five hours at 40°- 45°C. Hydrolysis can be carried out by single stage or two stage process. In single stage process, substrate is reacted with specific enzyme for a certain period of time at a specific pH and thereafter the reaction is stopped by heating the solution to deswtroy the enzyme. The two stage process is prefered to overcome the problem of bitter taste in casein hydrolysate. Here the casein solution is first digested using endopeptidase enzyme having high peptidase activity followed by using exopeptidase enzyme to remove residual bitter peptides and free amino acids. This process is used for commercial preparation of milk protein hydrolysate. The technological advances of protein hydrolysis have been helpful in improving solubility, emulsification, gelling, foaming and heat stability of resultant hydrolysates.

Protein hydrolysates are increasingly finding commercial applications in number of formulated foods. Diets suitable for geriatrics, high energy supplements, weight control diets, therapeutic and entric diets are some of the examples. The benefit of protein hydrolysis is for persons with impaired digestive functions and dietary allergies. Hydrolysis break down the protein into smaller peptides and amino acids are more easily available from pre digested proteins that allows faster intestinal absorption.

Buttermilk

Buttermilk is an important byproduct obtained during manufacture of butter. There are three types of buttermilk produced namely – sweet cream buttermilk which is obtained by churning pasteurized cream, sour buttermilk which is obtained by churning naturally sour cream and desi buttermilk which is obtained by churning dahi. It is estimated that nearly 3.2 million tones of butter is produced in India which is based on conversion of 6.5% of total milk production that goes for production of butter. An substantial amount is also produced during manufacture of desi butter (makkhan). This is called lassi or chhach and is generally consumed fresh or fed to animals. Buttermilk produced during manufacture of creamery butter made from pasteurized cream is called sweet cream buttermilk. It has similar composition as skim milk but contains higher concentration of phospholipids and fat globule membrane proteins. Till last few decades buttermilk solids were untapped until research focused on their role in health. The high nutritive value of buttermilk and concern for environmental pollution warrants its economical utilization. The differences in various physical and chemical properties of buttermilk and skim milk provide many choices for their attractive application in dairy product manufacture.

The chemical composition of buttermilk greatly varies depending on amount of water added during manufacturing of butter. On an average desi buttermilk contains about 4% total solids that comprises of 0.8% fat, 1.29% protein and 1.2% lactic acid. Sweet cream buttermilk contains around 9.0-9.5% total solids of which fat is 0.2-0.5%, protein 3.0-3.5%, lactose 4.5-4.8%, ash 0.6-0.7%. Buttermilk contains higher fat content than skim milk and is rich in phospholipids content. Buttermilk also contains higher proportion of protein mixture that comprises of milk fat globule membrane proteins. This protein is sloughed from the fat globule-milk-serum interface by churning process. The amount of milk fat globule membrane protein is however, not large in comparision to total buttermilk proteins. Phospholipids of buttermilk do not have short chain fatty acids. Principal fatty acids are palmitic and higher acids. The fatty acids of phospholipids contains 40% saturated fatty acids and the rest are non-conjugated di – penta un-saturated fatty acids. Phospholipids of buttermilk has more or less equal proportion of lecithin, cephalin, sphingomyelin with small portion of cerebrosides. Sweet cream buttermilk has lower acidity and curd tension but higher viscosity as compared to skim milk.

Table 8.4: Gross composition of buttermilk and skim milk

Constituents	Buttermilk	Skim milk
Total solids (%)	9.88	10.38
Fat (%)	0.59	0.05
Total protein (%)	3.73	4.27
Lactose (%)	4.81	5.20
Ash (%)	0.75	0.82
Phospholipids (mg%)	78.56	8.65
Titratable acidity (%LA)	0.12	0.16

Source: Gupta 2008

The composition of skim milk and sweet cream buttermilk are quite similar. Therefore, no problems are expected to encounter during normal processing adopted by most of the dairy factories. As a matter of fact the heat stability of buttermilk is considered to be better and therefore, making it more suitable to high heat treatments encountered during condensing and drying.

Uses of Buttermilk

Sour buttermilk, obtained from natural souring of milk / cream, is best converted into casein with slight modification in the processing conditions. Sweet cream buttermilk have been successfully used for standardization of whole milk for manufacture of market milk or paneer milk. Use of buttermilk for standardization of buffalo milk in preparation of tonned or standardized milk, improves palatability, heat stability, reduces curd tension without affecting keeping quality of final product. Standardizing whole milk with sweet cream buttermilk for preparation of paneer provides higher yield and good organoleptic quality with reasonable shelf life.

Sweet cream buttermilk may be used for preparation of variety of fermented and traditional dairy products like Yoghurt, dahi, channa, srikhand, soft cheeses etc. Sweet cream buttermilk has been used successfully for manufacture of cultured butter milk and lassi. Dahi obtained by admixture of whole milk and buttermilk provides softer body. It is suggested to incorporate 1-2% of skim milk powder for improving the body of dahi made from buttermilk. Similarly replacement of skim milk powder with buttermilk powder (upto 50%) have been used for manufacture of low fat yoghurt. This reduces the susceptibility of syneresis in yoghurt and dahi.

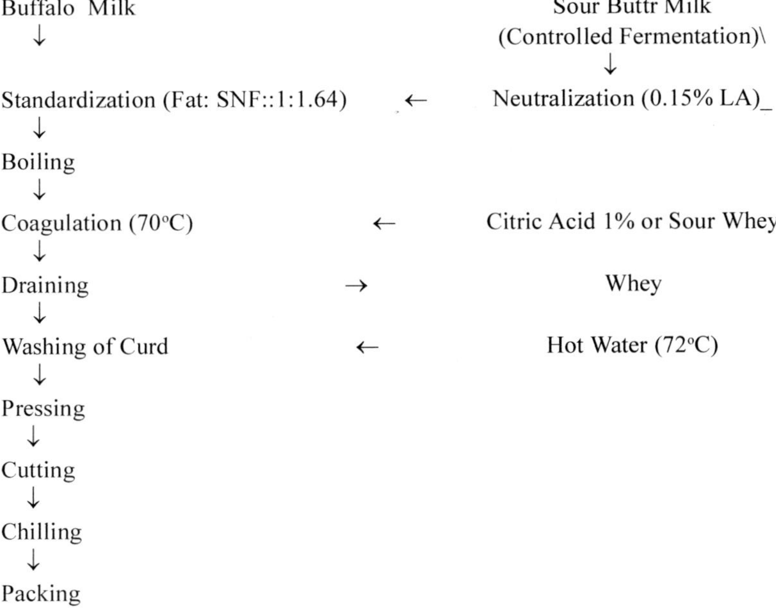

Fig. 8.3: Flow diagram of manufacturing paneer from sour butter milk

Channa produced from buffalo milk is generally harder and greasy. However, soft channa can be made from buffalo milk by admixing sweet cream buttermilk in the proportion of 60:100 (on total solid basis), adjusting fat and s.n.f. ratio to 1:2.1 and heating the mixture at 75°C and coagulating at pH 5.2.

In srikhand making, chakka obtained by draining whey from dahi, is an intermediate product. Use of buffalo milk produces hard and coarse texture of chakka. This can be improved by 50% replacement of skim milk with buttermilk to provide smooth body and texture. Dried buttermilk can replace skim milk powder in manufacture of gulabjamun mix powder. The high lecithin content in buttermilk may improve textural characteristics of rasogolla.

With growing awareness of dietary fat on human health, World wide research has been focused on development of low fat cheeses. Lowering fat content, lowers the content of fat globule membrane which effects the cheese texture and flavor. Incorporating 5% ultra filtered buttermilk in cheese milk may help to produce softer body and texture and higher yield during manufacture of reduced fat cheddar and mozzarella cheeses. Acceptable quality of cheddar cheese have been produced by admixing sweet cream buttermilk with buffalo milk with slight modification in processing techniques. Attempts have been made to substitute sweet cream buttermilk upto 75%, in place of water for adjusting moisture content in processed cheese.

As the composition of skim milk and buttermilk is nearly same and buttermilk having better heat stability, the conditions used for concentration and drying of skim milk can be adopted for drying of buttermilk. The most common utilization of sweet cream buttermilk is admixing with skim milk for purpose of drying. Admixture of buttermilk to skim milk produces skim milk powder having better solubility and low bulk density. However, the limit of admixing sweet cream buttermilk is to the tune of around 10%. Higher percentage may cause increase in the whey protein nitrogen (WPN) of the resultant powder. Generally in industry the sweet cream buttermilk is dried to produce buttermilk powder. The spray dried buttermilk powder is less free flowing and dusty. The high phospholipid content provides better oxidative stability to dried buttermilk.

Table 8.5: Characteristics of dried buttermilk and skim milk powders

Characteristics	Buttermilk powder	Skim milk powder
Moisture (%)	2.59	2.75
Fat (%)	6.38	1.05
Total protein (%)	37.09	40.28
Lactose (%)	47.01	48.20
Ash (%)	6.94	7.76
Phospholipids (mg%)	625.25	97.1
Titratable acidity (%LA)	1.17	1.39
Solubility index (ml)	0.15	0.30
Bulk density (g/ml)	0.345	0.544

Source : Gupta 2008

The dried buttermilk have several usage in formulating variety of general and health foods. The role of dried buttermilk solids in health foods is being investigated by many researchers. It has been reported that feeding of processed cheese containing 30% buttermilk concentrate to rats decreased total and low density lipoprotein cholesterol (LDL) content. Attempts have been made to isolate milk fat globule membrane material from buttermilk and skim milk retentate rich in phospholipids. Such isolates can be used as functional ingrediants in development of neutraceuticals. Buttermilk solids also demonstrate antioxidant properties and hence are suggested for use in stabilizing food matrix against lipid peroxidation. Judicious use of buttermilk solids in the development of functional foods is a promising area.

An important domestic beverage in India is "chacch or desi buttermilk" obtained by making desi butter at rural level. Usually salt or black pepper is added to chacch before direct consumption as a refreshing beverage. Lassi is yet another refreshing beverage made by mixing dahi with water, spices,salt or sugar. The consistency depends on ratio of dahi to water. Buttermilk solids can also be added in preparation of lassi. Salted lassi is widely relished in southern part of the country while sweetened lassi is popular in northern India. Buttermilk is also used for preparation of traditional products like Karhi, Raita or Rabadi, a fermented drink relished in the rural areas of Haryana state.

A large variety of beverages can be formulated using sweet cream buttermilk with addition of variety of rigion and climate specific fruits available throughout the country. Addition of fruit pulps or juices is an attractive aveneue for utilization of buttermilk solids. Incorporation of apple and leechi juice (30%), banana pulp (20%), guava pulp (10%) and mango pulp (20%) can be used for manufacture of acceptable quality refreshing beverage. Admixture of mango juice and buttermilk in the ratio of 20:80 have been used for the production of dried flavoured ready to reconstitute type drink.

World wide interest in probiotic foods has led to the development of variety of health drinks. Attempts have also been made to develop health promoting drinks from buttermilk by fermenting it with different probiotic organisms (various strains of Lactobacillus and Bifidobacteria genera). Such a drink has found to be helpful in reducing serum and liver cholesterol while increasing high density cholesterol.

These drinks have also been useful in controlling gut microbial status thereby reducing the incidence of diarrhea and other gut infections.

Ghee Residue

It is a brownish solid mass obtained as a byproduct of ghee manufacture. It contains considerable amounts of fat, protein and minerals. The colour of ghee residue may vary from light brown to dark brown, depending upon the heat treatment used during ghee making. It has smooth to granular texture with glossy exterior due to the presence of excessive free fat. It is estimated that about 33 percent of total milk produced in the country is diverted towards ghee making (Dairy India, 2007). About 30.4 million tones of ghee is, presently, manufactured in India. Taking the average yield of ghee residue as 1/10 th of the quantity of ghee produced, the amount of ghee residue work out to be more than 3 million tons per annum. The yield of ghee residue varies with the variation in the serum solid content of the raw material used. Ghee residue has soft smooth body but gets hardened, progressively, during storage. The textural characteristics changes fast, from smooth to hard and gritty. Ghee residue has an excellent source of natural flavouring compounds (carbonyls and lactones). It also contains natural antioxidants that may be helpful in controlling oxidation of lipids. The yield and chemical composition of ghee residue obtained from different sources of raw materials are provided in Table 8.6.

Table 8.6: Yield and chemical composition of ghee residue

Source	Yield (Kg/100kg)	Compositional constituents (%)				
		Moisture	Fat	Protein	Lactose	Ash
Indigenous butter (Makkhan)	1.60	13.40	33.40	32.80	15.40	5.20
Sweet cream	7.70	4.10	63.20	18.0	12.30	2.40
Sour cream	5.10	8.00	38.80	41.60	7.30	4.30
Washed sweet cream	3.50	1.70	80.80	16.20	Trace	1.30
Creamery butter	1.20	5.70	65.00	25.50	Trace	3.80

Source: Verma, 2002

Physico-chemical Properties of Ghee Residue

Particle size and density- Ghee is generally filtered using muslin cloth, for small scale or filter bags and centrifugal clarification for large scale manufacture. The average particle size (diameter) of ghee residue was found to be around 104.79 micron and the average density is about 1.14 g/sq. cm.

Lipids- Irrespective of the method of preparation of ghee, the lipids of ghee residue contain 53% lower chain fatty acids, 58.7% total saturated fatty acids, 41.3% un-saturated fatty acids. The polyunsaturated fatty acid content of ghee residue is about 4.4% higher than those in ghee. The lipids of ghee residue have lower Reichert and Polenske value, being 24.4 and 1.3 respectively, than that of ghee. It is also rich in phospholipids (1-9%). Most of the phospholipids remains in residue due to its polar nature. The content of phospholipids is dependent upon the method of preparation. It is highest in creamery butter method (17.39%) followed by desi butter method (4.95%) and least in direct creamery method (1.57%). Phospholipid content decreases as the period of heat treatment increases.

Proteins – Ghee residue usally have poor quality of proteins. The soluble nitrogen content decreases with heating time when cream or creamery butter method is employed for ghee making. Using paper chromatographic technique, one may detect about 11 free amino acids and 2 amines. These are expressed as mg of cystine hydrochloride/g and free sulphydryl content (μg/g) of ghee residue. Thye total reducing capacity of creamery butter ghee residue is 26 and free sulphydryl content is 2.9 μg/g. These substances were librated from protein during heat treatment and owing to their polar nature they are mostly retained in ghee residue. Whey protein (*β-lactoglobulin*) is the main source of sulphydryl compounds.

Milk sugars – Ghee residue obtained from ghee clarified at 120°C have been found to contain lactose (76.6 g), glucose (5.3 g) and galactose (14.1 g). As the period of heating is increased, the lactose content decreases with corresponding increase in galactose and glucose content. The unidentified sugars are found to increase as the period of heating is increased. This could be due to some breakdown products of sugar fragments formed during browning or caramelisation reactions.

Antioxidants – Ghee residue is a rich source of natural antioxidants. The overall antioxygenicpeoperties are due to both lipids and non-lipid constituents. The oxidative stability of ghee can be increased by increasing its phospholipids content by heat treatment process. Phospholipids in ghee residue shows maximum antioxidant activity as compared to alpha-tocopherol and vitamin A. Cephaline, among various phospholipid fractions, shows greatest antioxidant activity. Maximum transfer of phospholipid from ghee residue to ghee can be achieved by heating a mixture of ghee rtesidue and ghee in the ratio of 1:4 at 130°C. The antioxidant concentrate thus obtained can be added to ghee to give 0.1% phospholipid in ghee so as to increase its keepking quality. Higher temperature of clarification may decrease the antioxidant efficacy of ghee residue. Among non-lipid constituents certain amino acids (proline, cystine, tryptophane and lysine may contribute towards antioxidant property of ghee residue. Ghee residue also contain large amount of reducing substances including sulphydryl compounds that contribute to its antioxidant property. Ghee residue obtained from creamery butter method of ghee making has maximum antioxidant properties followed by ghee rsidueobtaine from desi butter and direct cream methods of ghee making. The natural antioxidant present in ghee residue is preferred than chemical/ synthetic antioxidents

Flavour compounds – Ghee residue is a rich source of natural flavouring compounds like free fatty acids, carbonyls and lactones. The level of these compounds in ghee residue is higher than those in ghee. Presence of these compounds, even in low levels, give ghee its characteristic flavour. Table 8.7 gives the concentration of potential flavouring compounds in ghee and ghee residue.

Table 8.7: Flavouring compounds in ghee & ghee residue

Flavouring compounds	Ghee	Ghee residue
FFA (μmol/g)	53.60	627.50
Carbonyles (μmol/g)	4.30	43.70
Lactones (μg/g)	30.30	3992.90

Source : Galhotra & Wadhawa,1993

Treatment and Processing

Just after manufacture, the ghee residue has soft and smooth body. However, during storage it progressively hardened. The textural changes are much faster during first 15 days of storage and by the end of month it becomes hard and gritty. If the ghee residue is intended for edible preparations it is necessary to process it so as to yield soft and smooth texture for its utilization. Various processing treatments have been suggested to keep the ghee residue soft viz. tying in the form of bundle and cooking in boiling water for 30 minutes, cooking in boiling 1% sodium bicarbonate, washing in 50% alcohol and then cooking in boiling water, washing in alcohol and them cooking in sodium bicarbonate solution etc. All these treatments make the residue soft and smooth. It helps to considerably reduce fat, lactose and acidity of the ghee residue and at the same time make the residue to absorb considerable amount of moisture. The keeping quality of treated ghee residue is about 1.5 to 2.0 months.

Recovery of fat from Ghee Residue

The dairy plants are more interested to recover as much ghee as possible from ghee residue. Generally ghee residue is mixed with hot water in ghee recovery vats. Here the water is heated so as to transfer occluded ghee of the residue to water it is then chilled to solidify the fat which is then recovered and mixed with next batch of clarification process. Alternatively, the hot water containing fat is centrifuged to recover the ghee. The method yields 25% ghee with 46% efficiency. Ghee can also be recovered by subjecting the hot residue to hydrolic pressure. This method gives the yield of 45% with 67% efficiency. This is an economical, simple, practical and efficient method requiring no electricity or sophisticated equipments.

Applications of Ghee Residue

Ghee residue being rich source of fat and proteins is a valuable material for human dietary supplement. The physico-chemical properties of processed ghee residue make it suitable for certain confectionary usage. Ghee residue by virtue of its chemical composition, bulk production, physical characteristics, longer shelf life has great potential for exploiting its utilization in food industry.

1. ***Candy preparation*** – Ghee residue can well be used for preparation of candy type product. The preparation requires 1.0 kg processed ghee residue which is mixed with 50% sugar syrup and excess of moisture evaporated over slow fire with continuous stirring. When the mass is sufficiently sticky about 200g of coconut powder is added. The contents is spread on the tray and allowed to cool. Then it is cut into small cubes and rapped in parchment paper.
2. ***Bufi type confection*** – Before using ghee residue in khoa, it was treated with 0.5% sodium bicarbonate for 30 minutes. The processed ghee residue was then mixed with khoa in the ratio of 1:1(total solid basis) and sugar @ 75% of total solids. the mass was heated with vigorous stirring for 10-15 minutes. Two third of this mixture was spread into well greased tray. To the remaining 1/3 rd mass chocolate powder was added @ 8% of total solids and mixed well. This was applied over the first layer in the tray and allowed to cool at room temperature and cut into uniform size and shape.
3. ***Bakery product*** – Sponge cake and nan-khatai type (cookie) products can be made from processed ghee residue obtained from ripened cream. For these products the part of vegetable oil used for their preparation was replaced with ghee residue fat. Almost 30% of vegetable oil for cookies and 20% for cake can be replaced. Incorporation of ghee residue upto 30% into cookies dough increased the spread factor and improved the flavour of resultant cookie.

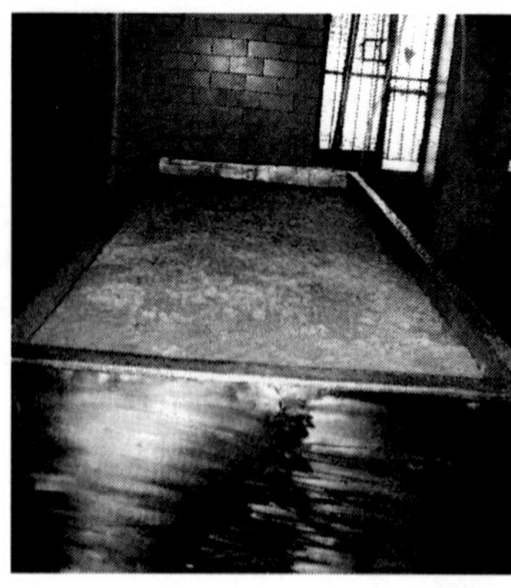
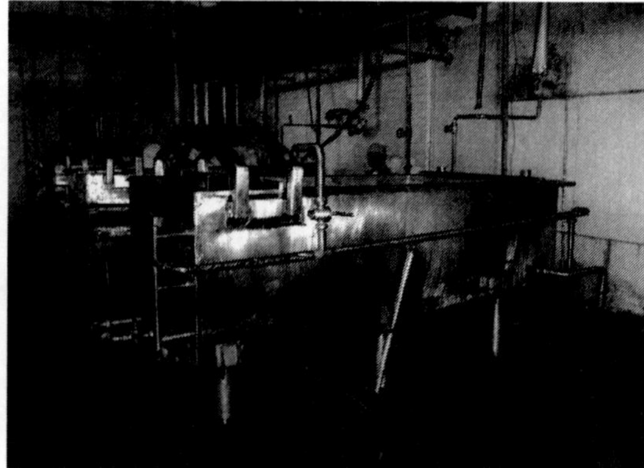

Fig. 8.1: Fat recovery tank

Preparation of chocolate – To prepare chocolate 1.0 kg of processed ghee rsidue is added with 50% sugar syrup and mixed thoroghly. The contenta are dessicated over slow fire till dough is formed. At this stage cocoa powder (500 g) and skim milk powder (70 g) are added and stirred vigorously till pat is formed. This is then spread on a plate and cooled overnight, cut into cubes or slabs and wrapped in parchment paper. The produst has shelf life of more than three months.

Suggested Readings

Boopathy, R. (1994) Enzyme technology in food and health industries. Indian Food Industry, 34:22-37.

Corredig, M., Roesch, R.R. and Delgleish, D.G. (2003) Production of novel ingrediants from buttermilk. J. Dy. Sci., 86(9):2744-2750.

El-Sayed, M.S., Hamed, I.M., Asker, A.A., Hamzawi, L.F. and El-Sayed, M.M. (2006) Plasma lipid profile of rats fed with processed cheese spread enriched with buttermilk concentrate. Egyp.J. Dairy Sci., 34(2):43-60.

El-Shafei, K. (2003) Production of probiotic cultured buttermilk using mixed culture. Egyp.J.Dairy Sci., 31(1):43-60.

Galhotra, K.K. and Wadhawa, B.K. (1993) Chemistry of ghee residue, its significance and utilization. Indian J Dairy Science, 46: 142-146.

Gokhale, A.J., Pandya, A.J. and Upadhyay, K.G. (1999) Effect of substitution of water with sweet cream buttermilk on quality of processed cheese spread. Ind.J.Dairy Sci., 52(4):256-261.

Gupta, V.K. (2000) Enzymic production of protein hydrolysate for food application.

Gupta, V.K. (2008) Development In the manufacturing technology of casein products. Technological advances in utilization of dairy by products. Lecture compendium, CAS in Dairy Technology, NDRI, Karnal.

Muller, L.L. (1982) Manufacture of casein, caseinate and co-precipitate. In: Developments in dairy chemistry. P.F.Fox (ed) Vol., 1:328-330.

New concept in dairy technology. Lecture compendium, CAS in Dairy Technology, NDRI, Karnal.

Panyam, D. and Kilara, A. (1996) Enhancing functionality of food protein by enzymic modification. J. Food Sci. Technol., 7:120-125.

Rao, H.G..R. and Kumar, A.H. (2005) Spray drying of mango juice-buttermilk blends. Lait. 85(4/5):395-404.

Rodas, B.A., Angulo, J.O., Cruz, j. De-La and Gracia, H.S. (2002) Preparation of probiotic buttermilk with *L.reuteri*. Milchwissenschaft, 57(1):26-28.

Santha, I.M. and Narayanan, K.M. (1978) Composition of ghee residue lipids. Indian J Dairy Science, 31(4):365-369.

Shreshtha, R.G. and Gupta S.K. (1979) Dahi from sweet cream buttermilk. Indian Dairyman, 31: 657-660.

Shukla, F.C., Sharma, A. and Singh, B. (2004) Preparation of fruit beverage using whey and buttermilk. J. Fd. Sci. Technol. 41(1):102-105.

Southward, C.R. (1989) Uses of casein and casienates. In: Developments in Dairy Chemistry-4, P.A. Fox (Ed), Elsevier Science Publication Ltd. England. P. 173-244.

Southward, C.R. (1994) Utilisation of milk component casein. In: Modern Dairy Technology. Vol.1 Advances in milk processing. R.K.Robinson (ed) 2nd edition, Chapman Hall, U.K. pp 375-432.

Wong, P.Y.Y. and Kitts, D.D. (2003) Chemistry of buttermilk solids antioxidant activity. J. Dairy Sci., 86(5):1541-1547.

9

Food Regulatory and Quality Assurance Aspects

Over the past several years, there has been significant change in consumer perception on quality and food safety. Consumers are demanding healthy, nutritious and cost-effective products processed under controlled hygienic conditions. Food safety concern, in recent years, has become dominant and important. The requirement of food safety and quality assurance has never been so demanding as it is now. Globally food safety is being addressed independent of food quality. In anticipation of consumer demands on food safety, food sanitary standards at national and international levels are under constant review. Several inter governmental agencies/organizations are engaged in work related to quality assurance and food safety. Amongst these World Health Organization (WHO) and Codex Alimentarius Commission (CAC) play the major role in protecting public health and defining standards of quality and safety aspects of foods for regional and or world wide usage.

Regulatory Institutions

The quality environment in the Indian food processing sector revolves around compulsory legislation which specify minimum standard and certification system. Legal standards are generally made to have control over the quality of foods offered for sale and to safeguard the consumer from health hazards posed by practice of adulteration. There are basically three types of Indian standards namely.

Food Safety and Standard Act 2006

Food processing industry in India is presently governed by large number of food laws and/ or orders which are administrated by various ministries and are not considered condusive for effective fixation of food standard and their enforcement. The multiplicity of laws leads to greater confusion for investors, manufacturers, traders and consumers alike. Need for therefore felt for integration of such laws for effectively regulating the food quality. The food safety and standard act was passed by the parliament with the objective of ensuring safe food to the consumers. The act has 12 chapters, 101 clauses and 2 schedules. The major objectives of the act are :-

a) To provide single window system for matters related to standards and regulations.

b) Shifting emphasis from PFA to broader concept of food safety and management system.

c) Formulation of standards, samples, analysis, labelling under scientific advice.

d) Regulating manufacture, storage, distribution and sale to promote global trade.

e) Rationalize and strengthen existing enforcement mechanisms.

f) Providing graded civil and criminal penalties for food safety violations.

The Ministry of Health and Family Welfare, Government of India has recently announced "Food Safety and Standard Rule 2011" through Gezette of India Extraordinary Part II and III dated 19th January 2011. These rules are applicable and in force from 5th August 2011 all over India. The food safety and standard authority will be the supreme body to look into implementation and regulation of this act. The authority will consist of 7 members from different ministries (agriculture, commerce, health, food processwing, small scale industries, legislative and consumers affairs); 2 from food industry; 3 food technologist/ scientists; 2 representatives from consumer organisation; 5 representatives from state; 2 representatives of farmers and 1 representatives from retailer organisation. The authority will have central advisory committee, scientific panels and scientific committee for providing scientific opinions. The state Govt. shall appoint commissioner of food safety for effective enforcement of requirements laid down in this act, rules and regulations made there under. The second schedule of the act repeals all other existing acts and orders except

MMPO 1992. Central and state Govts. will establish appellate tribunal which will look into the matters related to violation of this act.

Bureau of Indian Standards (BIS)

BIS is a statutory body established under the Ministry of Consumers Affair in 1986. It is the national standard organisation of India. It is responsible for laying down the Indian standards in consultation with the experts drawn from manufacturing units, research and technical institutions, purchase organisations and other concern parties. It deals in formulation of standards in processed food sector and implementation through voluntary and third party certification systems. These standards cover raw material permitted, their quality parameters, hygiene conditions of manufacturing, packaging and labelling requirements and are amended suitably from time to time. Manufacturers complying with these standards can obtain "ISI" or "BIS" certification and exhibit the same on their product package. In BIS standards, more emphasis is laid on the microbiological requirements. The standards are primarily focused on food processing establishments. Recently, the Bureau has launched a quality management system certification scheme to help strengthen the industry for their quality control programme. BIS operates following certification schemes:

- BIS product certification scheme.
- Quality scheme certification as per IS/ISO 9000 series.
- Environmental management system as per IS/ISO 14000 series.
- Hazard analysis and critical control point (HACCP) as per ISO-15000.
- BIS has also started ECOMARK scheme for environmental friendly products. This was launched for protection of environment and ecology.

AGMARK Standard

These standards are formulated by the Directorate of Marketing and Inspection, under Ministry of Agriculture, Govt. Of India. It enforces the Agriculture Produce (Grading and Marketing) act which was first enacted in 1937. Under this act, grade standards are prescribed for agricultural and allied commodities. These are known as "AGMARK" standards. It categorises the commodities into various grades such as – special and standard. Grading under this act is voluntary and manufacturers who comply with the standards laid down in DMI are allowed to use "AGMARK" logo on their products. "AGMARK" gives the consumers an assurance of quality in accordance with the standards laid down. However, these standards are not mandatory. Presently, three dairy products namely: Ghee, Butter and dairy spreads are graded under this scheme.

Product Definitions and Standards

Cream : Including sterilised cream means the product of cow or buffalo milk or combination thereof. It shall be free from starch and other ingredients foreign to milk. It may be of following three categories, namely:

Low fat cream : containing milk fat not less than 25% by weight.

Medium fat cream : containing milk fat not less than 40% by weight.

High fat cream : containing milk fat not less than 60% by weight.

Note : Cream sold without any indication about milk fat content shall be treated as high fat cream.

Malai means the product rich in butterfat prepared by boiling and cooling cow or buffalo milk or a combination therefore. It shall contain not less than 25% milk fat.

Cream Powder means the product obtained by partial removal of water from cream obtained from milk of cow and/or buffalo. The fat and/or protein content of the cream may be adjusted by addition and/or withdrawal of milk constituents in such a way as not to alter the whey protein to casein ratio of the milk being adjusted. It shall be of uniform colour and shall have pleasant taste and flavour free from off flavour and rancidity. It shall also be free from vegetable oil/ fat, mineral oil, added flavour and any substance foreign to milk. The product may contain food additives permitted in these regulations including Appendix A. It shall conform to the microbiological requirements prescribed in Appendix B. It shall conform to the following requirements:

(i) Moisture not more than 5.0 percent

(ii) Milk fat not less than 42.0 percent

(iii) Milk protein in Milk solid fat not less than 34.0 percent

Butter means the fatty product derived exclusively from milk of Cow and/or Buffalo or its products principally in the form of an emulsion of the type water-in-oil. The product may be with or without added common salt and starter cultures of harmless lactic acid and/or flavour producing bacteria. Table butter shall be obtained from pasteurised milk and/ or other milk products which have undergone adequate heat treatment to ensure microbial safety. It shall be free from animal, body fat, vegetable oil and fat, mineral oil and added flavour. It shall have pleasant taste and flavour free from off flavour and rancidity. It may contain food additives permitted in these Regulations including Appendix A. It shall conform to the microbiological requirements prescribed in Appendix B. Provided that where butter is sold or offered for sale without any indication as to whether it is table or desi butter, the standards of table butter shall apply.

It shall conform to the following requirements:

Table butter : Moisture-16.0 percent m/m, Milk Fat-80.0 percent m/m, Milk solids- Not more than 1.5 percent and Common salt- not more than 3.0 percent.

Cooking butter : Milk Fat-76.0 percent m/m.

Fat spread means a product in the form of water in oil emulsion, of an aquous phase and a fat phase of edible oils and fats excluding animal body fats. The individual oil and fat used in the spread shall conform to the respective standards prescribed by these regulations. Fat spread shall be classified into the following three groups :-

(a) ***Milk fat spread*** : Fat content will be exclusively milk fat.

(b) ***Mixed fat spread*** : Fat content will be a mixture of milk fat with any one or more of hydrogenated, unhydrogenated refined edible vegetable Oils or interesterified fat.

(c) ***Vegetable fat spread*** : Fat content will be a mixture of any two or more of hydrogenated, unhydrogenated refined edible vegetable Oils or interesterified fat.

It may 'contain' edible common salt not exceeding 2 percent by weight in aqueous phase; milk solid not fat: It may contain food additives permitted in these Regulations and Appendices. It shall be free from animal body fat, mineral oil and wax. Vegetable fat spread shall contain raw or refined Sesame oil (Til oil) in sufficient quantity so that when separated fat is mixed with refined groundnut oil in the proportion of 20:80 the red colour produced by Baudouin test shall not be lighter than 2.5 red units in 1 cm cell on a Lovibond scale. It shall also conform to the following standards, namely:— Fat not more than 80 percent and not less than 40 percent by weight. Moisture not more than 56 percent and not less than 16 percent by weight. Melting point of extracted fat not more than 37°C (capillary slip method) in case of vegetable fat spread. Unsaponifiable matter of extracted fat (a) In case of milk fat and mixed fat spread not more than 1 percent by weight (b) In case of vegetable fat spread not more than 1.5 percent. Acid value of extracted fat not more than 0.5. The vegetable fat spread shall contain not less than 25 IU synthetic vitamin 'A' per gram at the time of packing and shall show a positive test for vitamin 'A' when tested by Antimony Trichloride (Carr-Price) reagents (as per I.S. 5886 - 1970)". It shall contain Starch not less than 100 ppm and not mor than 150 ppm. The fat content shall be declared on the label. In mixed fat spread, the milk fat content shall also be declared on the label along with the total fat content. The word 'butter' will not be associated while labelling the product.

It shall be compulsorily sold in sealed packages weighing not more than 500g. under Agmark certificate mark.

Table margarine means an emulsion of edible oils and fats with water. It shall be free from rancidity, mineral oil and animal body fats. It may contain common salt not exceeding 2.5 percent, skimmed milk powder not exceeding 2 percent; it may contain food additives permitted in these Regulations and Appendices. It shall conform to the following specifications, namely - Fat not less than 80 percent (m/m). Moisture not less than 12 percent and not more than 16 percent (m/m). Vitamin A not less than 30IU per gram, of the product at the time of sale. Melting point of extracted fat 31°C to 37°C (Capillary Slip Method). Unsaponifiable matter not more than 1.5 percent by weight of extracted fat. Free fatty acids (as oleic acid) of extracted fat not more than 0.25 percent by weight OR Acid Value not more than 0.5 It shall contain not less than 5.0 percent of its weight of Til oil but sufficient to ensure that when separated fat is mixed with refined groundnut oil in the proportion of 20:80 the red colour produced by the Baudouin test shall not be lighter than 2.5 red units in 1 cm cell on a lovibond scale. Provided that such coloured and flavoured margarine shall also contain starch not less than 100 ppm and not more than 150 ppm. Provided further, that such coloured and flavoured margarine shall only be sold in sealed packages weighing not more than 500gms. Test for Argemone oil shall be negative.

Bakery and Industrial Margarine means an emulsion of vegetable oil product with water. It shall be free from added colour and flavour, rancidity, mineral oil and animal body fats. It may contain common salt not exceeding 2.5 percent. However, it may contain food additives permitted in these Regulations and

Appendices. It shall conform to the following standards, namely:–Fat not less than 80 percent m/m. Moisture not less than 12 percent and not more than 16 percent m/m. The separated fat of the products shall conform to the following: – Vitamin A not less than 30 IU per gram at the time of packaging and shall show a positive test for Vitamin 'A' when tested by Antimony trichloride (carrprice) reagents (as per IS 5886-1970). Melting point by 31°C-41°C Capillary slip method. Unsaponifiable matter not exceeding 2.0 percent but in case of the products where proportion of Rice bran oil is more than 30 percent by wt. the unsaponifiable matter shall be not more than 2.5 percent by wt. provided quantity of Rice bran oil is declared on the label of such product as laid down in Regulation 2.4.5 (34) of Food Safety and Standards (Food Products Standards and Food Additive) Regulations, 2011. Free Fatty Acid Not more than 0.25 percent. calculated as Oleic Not more than 0.5. acid or Acid value. It shall contain raw or refined sesame oil (Til oil) in sufficient quantity so that when the product is mixed with refined groundnut oil in the proportion of 20 : 80, the colour produced by the Boudouin test shall not be lighter than 2.0 red unit in a 1 cm. cell on a Lovibond scale. Test for argemone oil shall be negative.

Ghee means the pure clarified fat derived solely from milk or curd or from desi (cooking) butter or from cream to which no colouring matter or preservative has been added. The standards of quality of ghee produced in a State or Union Territory shall be as follows – Moisture (Max.)- 0.5%, BR value- 40.0 to 43.0,RM value-24 – 28 and FFA as oleic acid (max.)- 3.0 Percent. Baudouin test shall be negative. However, for cotton tract areas these values may be as follows - BR value- 41.5 to 45.0, RM value-21-26 and FFA as oleic acid (max.) -3.0 Percent.

By cotton tract is meant the areas in the States where cotton seed is extensively fed to the cattle and so notified by the State Government concerned.

Butter oil and Anhydrous Milk fat/Anhydrous Butter oil means the fatty products derived exclusively from milk and/or products obtained from milk by means of process which result in almost total removal of water and milk solids not fat. It shall have pleasant taste and flavour free from off odour and rancidity. It shall be free from vegetable oil/ fat, animal body fat, mineral oil, added flavour and any other substance foreign to milk. It may contain food additives permitted in these regulations including Appendix A. It shall conform to the microbiological requirements prescribed in Appendix B. It shall conform to the following requirements:— B.R reading at 40°C-40-44°C, Moisture m/m Not more than 0.4 percent and Not more than 0.1 percent for *Anhydrous Butter*

Oil, Milk Fat m/m Not less than 99.6 percent and Not less than 99.8 percent for *Anhydrous Butter Oil*, Reichert Value Not less than 24, F.F.A as oleic acid Not more than 0.4 percent and Not more than 0.3 percent for *Anhydrous Butter Oil,* Peroxide Value (milli eqvt of Oxygen/ Kg fat)- Not more than 0.6 percent and Not more than 0.3 percent for *Anhydrous Butter Oil*, Boudouins Test shall be Negative.

Analytical Techniques for Quality Assurance

Analysis of unsalted (cooking) butter and table butter

Tests are performed on table/cooking butter to have control over meeting the legal standards prescribed by FSSAI with respect to minimum fat content and maximum moisture, curd and salt content.

Sampling

Remove several plugs from the outside to the center of the butter block and collect in a container. Mix the contents into a uniform mass. Pack it into a screw cap bottle and keep in freezer until use.

Determination of Moisture

Requirements : Aluminium butter cup, tong, hot plate, dessicator, conical flask, balance, burette, etc.

Procedure : Take weight of empty butter cup. Weigh 10g of well mixed sample in butter cup. Heat the contents over hot plate with constant circular motion. Continue heating until foaming has ceased and the curd has attained golden brown colour. Allow the cup to cool in dessicator. Weigh the cup. Calculate moisture percentage from the differences in weights.

Calculation: Percent Moisture = B – C/B – A x 100

Where, A = Weight of empty cup

B = Weight of empty cup + sample

C = Weight of cup after heating

Determination of Curd and Salt

Requirements : Aluminium dish, tong, hot plate, desiccators, balance, petroleum ether

Procedure : Add 10 – 15ml of petroleum ether in the above butter cup and mix well. Allow to stand for settling of curd. Decant the ether layer into aluminium dish. Repeat extraction twice and collect ether layers by decanting. Dry the cup contents over a hot plate to dryness. Cool and weigh the cup.

Calculation:- Percent curd + salt = D – A/B – A x 100

Where, A = Weight of empty cup

B = Weight of empty cup + sample

D = Weight of cup after heating

Determination of Salt

Requirements : Conical flask, burette, beaker, water bath, potassium chromate indicator, 0.1N silver nitrate and calcium carbonate.

Procedure : Weigh 5 g of well mixed sample, from above cup, into 250 ml conical flask. Add 100ml of boiling distilled water, swirl the contents and allow to stand for 10 minutes. Add 2 ml of potassium chromate indicator and 0.25 g calcium carbonate. Mix the contents and titrate against 0.1N silver nitrate solution until brick red colour persist for half minutes. Carry out blank without sample.

Calculation : Percent salt = 5.85 x N x (V1 – V2)/W

Where, N = Normality of silver nitrate solution.

V1 = Volume of silver nitrate used for sample titration

V2 = Volume of silver nitrate used for blank titration

W = Weight of sample

Fat percent = 100 – (moisture + curd + salt)

Curd percent = (curd + salt) - Salt

Analysis of Table Spreads

1. Total fat

Requirements : Rose-Gottleib tube/Majonnier flask, fat evaporating dish, rubber stoppers, ammonia solution, diethyl ether, petroleum ether, ethyl alcohol, centrifuge machine, hot plate, oven, desiccator, weighing balance (electronic-top loading)

Procedure : Weigh 2-4 g of well-mixed sample in a beaker. Add 3 ml of 20% HCl solution and mix well. Transfer contents into extraction flask. Add 10 ml of alcohol and again mix well. Add 25 ml of diethyl ether, stopper the tube with cork and shake vigorously for one minute. Remove the cork and add 25 ml of petroleum ether, stopper and shake well for 30 seconds. Allow the tube to stand until ethereal layer is separated clearly from the aqueous layer (for Rose-Gottlieb method). In case of Majonnier method- centrifuge the Majonnier flask for 10 minutes. Decant the clear ethereal layer into a previously weighed aluminium fat dish. Repeat extraction with 15 ml portions each of diethyl ether and petroleum ether, twice to completely extract fat from the sample. Transfer the ethereal layers from each extraction into the fat dish. Place the fat dish on a hot plate (60°-65° C) and allow the ether layer to evaporate slowly. Dry the residual fat at 125° C in an oven for 1 hour and then allow the fat dish to cool by placing in a desiccators. Weigh the fat dish and note the weight. Repeat heating, cooling and weighing until successive weighing do not differ by more than 1 mg. Calculate amount of fat by difference of weight in fat dish before and after extraction (reading A). Divide reading A by the weight of sample and multiply by 100 to get percent fat in sample.

Calculation: Percent fat = (Wt. Of residue/Wt. Of sample) x 100

2. Moisture Test

Requirements : Moisture dish, Desiccators, hot air oven, weighing balance.

Procedure : Weigh accurately a clean and dry empty dish (A).Transfer 3-5 g of sample into the dish and note the weight (B).Place the dish on hot plate and allow the water to evaporate. Place the dish in hot air oven at 105° C for 1 hours.

Transfer the dish to a desiccator and allow cooling for 30 minutes. Weigh the contents and note the weight (C). Repeat heating and cooling until difference in two successive weights do not exceed 0.5 mg.

Observations

Weight of empty dish = A g

Weight of empty dish + sample = B g

Weight of dish after drying = C g

Calculations

Weight of sample (X) = Reading B – Reading A

Weight after drying (Y) = Reading C – Reading A

Percent moisture = B – C/B - A x 100

3. Salt Content

Requirements **:** Conical flask, burette, beaker, water bath, potassium chromate indicator, 0.1N silver nitrate and calcium carbonate.

Procedure : Weigh 5g of well mixed sample, from above cup, into 250ml conical flask. Add 100ml of boiling distilled water, swirl the contents and allow to stand for 10 minutes. Add 2ml of potassium chromate indicator and 0.25g calcium carbonate. Mix the contents and titrate against 0.1N silver nitrate solution until brick red colour persist for half minutes. Carry out blank without sample.

Calculation : Percent salt = 5.85 x N x (V1 – V2) / W

Where, N = Normality of silver nitrate solution.

V1 = Volume of silver nitrate used for sample titration.

V2 = Volume of silver nitrate used for blank titration.

W = Weight of sample.

4. Unsaponifiable Matter and Acid Value

When fat is saponified with excess of alkali soap is formed and unsaponified matter is released. It consist of sterols, tocopherol and vitamin A etc. These can be extracted from saponified fat and can be estimated gravimetrically. Acidity of fat is because of the presence of free fatty acids and is an index of lypolytic rancidity, that effects shelf life of fat rich products. The estimation is based on acid-base titration and is expressed as % oleic acid.

Fat extraction : Weigh about 10-20 g of sample (Table spread) into a beaker. Add 25-30 ml of hot distilled water and mix well. Transfer the contents to 250 ml separating funnel. Add 25 ml of 95% ethyl alcohol and shake well. Subsequently, add 60 ml of petroleum ether and 40 ml of ethyl ether. Shake the contents well. Allow to stand undisturbed for few minutes. Decant the solvent in a tared aluminium dish. Allow the ether to evaporate at 45°-50°C over a hot plate. Use the extracted fat for further analysis.

(a) Determination of Unsaponifiable matter : Draw 5g sample of extracted fat into saponification flask. Add 50 ml of alcoholic KOH and reflex for one hour.

Transfer the contents into 500 ml separating funnel. Rinse the flask first with 100-150 ml distilled water followed rinsing with ethyl ether. Transfer all washings to separating funnel. Mix the contents gently and allow to stand for 5-10 minutes.

Collect aqueous layer in same saponification flask and ether layer into conical flask. Make two more extractions using 2x50 ml ether portions and collect aqueous and ether layer as before. Transfer the ether layer into separating funnel and wash with 3x20 ml portions of distilled water and 3x20 ml portions of aqueous solution of 0.5N KOH alternatively. Discard aqueous layer after each washing. Wash excess of alkali with distilled water until wash water is alkali free.

Filter the contents through Whatman filter paper No. 4 with anhydrous sodium sulphate to remove traces of water. Collect the filtrate in a pre-weighed flask and evaporate ether to dryness over a steam water bath or hot plate. Transfer the flask in an oven maintained at 80° C for 10 minutes. Cool in desiccators and weigh the residue.

Calculation : Unsaponifiable matter (% by weight) = (W/m) x 100

Where W = Weight of residue

m = Weight of sample

(b) Determination of acid value : Weigh 5g sample of extracted fat in a 250 ml conical flask. Take 25 ml of neutral alcohol in another flask and heat the contents to boiling, while still hot, neutralize the contents using 0.1N NaOH.

Mix the contents of two flasks and bring it to boil. While still hot , titrate against standard aqueous solution of alkali (NaOH), using phenolphthalein as indicator.

Note: the volume of NaOH used for titration.

Calculation : Acid value = (5.61 x V) / W

Where V = Volume of standard alkali used for titration.

W = Weight of sample

(c) Phytosterol test : Weigh 5g sample of extracted fat in a 250 ml conical flask. Add 10 ml of 1% alcoholic digitonine solution. Allow the contents to cool in refrigerator for 12 hours. Filter the contents through Whatman No 1 filter paper in buchner funnel.

Collect the precipitate of sterol digitonine and wash with cold water until foaming stops. Wash with 25 ml of alcohol and diethyl ether respectively. Dry the filter paper in an oven at 102° C for 10-15 minutes. Collect the dry precipitate (residue) and note the weight.

Calculation : Percent total sterol = (0.25 x P/ W) 100

Where P = Weight of precipitate(residue)

W = Weight of sample

Analysis of Ghee, Butter-oil and Anhydrous Butter-oil

Fats and oils exhibit certain physical and chemical characteristics. The nature, proportion and manner of distribution of glycerol esters determine character of fat type. Milk fat has specific fat constants which are different than other fats. The tests are helpful in detecting adulterations and to maintain legal standards.

Moisture Test

Requirements : Moisture dish, Desiccators, hot air oven, weighing balance.

Procedure : Weigh accurately a clean and dry empty dish.(A)Transfer 10 g of sample into the dish and note the weight (B). Place the dish on hot plate and allow the water to evaporate. Place the dish in hot air oven at 105° C for 1 hours.

Transfer the dish to a desiccator and allow cooling for 30 minutes. Weigh the contents and note the weight. (C). Repeat heating and cooling until difference in two successive weights do not exceed 0.5 mg.

Observations

Weight of empty dish = A g

Weight of empty dish + sample = B g

Weight of dish after drying = C g

Calculations

Weight of sample (X) = Reading B – Reading A

Weight after drying (Y) = Reading C – Reading A

Percent moisture = B – C/B - A x 100

Free Fatty Acid (FFA) or Acidity

Acidity in ghee is expressed as percentage of free fatty acid calculated as Oleic acid as it is the main component of FFA. The maximum permissible limit is 3.0%.

(a) Titration Method

Requirements : Beaker, flask, N/10 NaOH, alcohol, burette, Phenolphthalein indicator.

Procedure : Weigh ~10 g of sample in a conical flask. Add 50 ml of neutral alcohol and boil the contents. Add few drops of indicator and titrate the contents, while boiling, using N/10 NaOH to pink color end point. Note volume of NaOH used. Express result in % free fatty acid (FFA).

Calculation

% FFA = Vol. of NaOH used x 28.2/9/wt. of sample

(b) Colorimetric Method

Requirements : Beaker, Conical flask, Centrifuge tubes (15 ml), Clinical centrifuge, colorimeter.

Reagents : Cupric acid pyridine (CAP) reagent adjusted to pH 6.0-6.2, Benzene.

Preparation of standard curve

Stock solution : Dissolve 6.34ml of pure Oleic acid in 100 ml benzene.

Working solution : Pipette out 1 ml of stock solution in a 100 ml volumetric flask and make up the volume with benzene.

Pipette 0.5: 1.0; 1.5, 2.0, 2.5, 3.0 and 3.5 ml of working solution in marked centrifuge tubes. Add 2.0 ml of CAP reagent in all the tubes, stopper and shake contents vigorously. Centrifuge at 5000 rpm for 5 minutes.

Take supernatant and observe optical density (OD) in a colorimeter using red filter. Adjust colorimeter to 0.0 OD with benzene. Draw a graph between micromoles concentration and optical density.

Procedure : Weigh accurately 5.0g of fat in 25 ml volumetric flask and makeup the volume with benzene. Take 1.0 ml of this solution in a glass stoppered centrifuge tube. Add 2.0 ml of CAP reagent and 9.0 ml of benzene. Shake vigorously and centrifuge at 5000 rpm for 5 minutes. Take supernatant and observe optical density as for standard curve. Plot the reading in standard graph and find out the concentration of FFA in sample. Multiply the reading with 250 to calculate percent FFA in the sample.

Butyro Refractometer Reading (B.R. Value)

Requirements : Beaker, glass rod, butyrorefractometer, water bath.

Procedure : Melt the sample at 40° C. Place one drop of sample onto butyrorefractometer lens. Maintain temperature at 40° C by circulating hot water through the water bath. Observe the reading on instrument scale directly and make note.

The BR reading for milk fat should be in the range of 40-43.

Reichert-Meissl Value (RM Value)

It is defined as the number of milliliters of 0.1 N aqueous alkali solution required to neutralize the water soluble steam volatile fatty acids distilled from 5.0g of fat under precise conditions.

Requirements : RM flask, burrett, pipette, measuring cylinder, funnel, filter paper, distil head, burner., distillation apparatus.

Reagents : Glycerol (98%), NaOH (50%), N/9 NaOH solution, ethyl alcohol, dilute sulphuric acid (40 ml to neutralize 2 ml of 50% NaOH), phenolphthalein indicator (0.5%).

Procedure : Weigh ~5g of sample in a Reichert-Meissl flask. Add 20g glycerol and 2 ml of 50% NaOH. Heat the contents with stirring till the liquid is cleared and cool the contents to room temperature. Add 93 ml of boiled distilled water before the soap is solidified. Add few pieces of glass beads followed by 50 ml of diluted sulphuric acid and immediately connect the flask with distillation apparatus. Heat the contents, without boiling, until insoluble acids are completely melted. Increase the flame and start distillation and collect 110 ml of the distillate within 20 minutes in a marked flask.Remove the flask containing distillate and discontinue heating. Cool the distillate to 15° C for 10 minutes using ice cold water. Mix the contents and filter through Whatman No. 4 filter paper, reject first few drops and collect 100 ml filtrate. Titrate the filtrate with N/9 NaOH using phenolphthalein as indicator. Carry out blank in the same manner.

Calculation

6.11 x vol. of NaOH used / wt. of sample

Peroxide Value (PV)

It is an index of oxidative rancidity and is defined as number of milliliters of 0.002 N sodium thiosulphate required to neutralize the iodine librated from 1.0 g of fat. It is expressed in terms of mill moles.

Requirements : Conical flask, rubber stopper with hole, balance, burette, water bath and pipette.

Reagents : Acetic acid – chloroform solvent mixture (2:1), 0.002 N sodium thiosulphste, 1% starch solution (freshly prepared).

Procedure : Weigh accurately 1.0 + 0.01g of sample in 150 ml conical flask. Add 20.ml of solvent mixture and heat the contents on boiling water bath for 30 seconds. Cool to room temperature and add 30 ml distilled water. Titrate against 0.002 N sodium thiosulphate solution using starch as indicator.

Calculation : Divide the volume of sodium thiosulphate used with the weight of sample to get PV.

Total Cholesterol

Declaration of total cholesterol content of ghee samples have now become mandatory to be displayed on the package as nutritional facts and hence, its determination has become important under new Indian food safety law, 2011.

Requirements: Conical flask, glass test tubes, glass stopper, balance, spectrophotometer/ colorimeter, water bath and pipette.

Reagents : Liebergmann-Burchard (LB) reagent – Mix 1.0ml of concentrated sulphuric acid in chilled 20.0ml acetic anhydride and keep solution at 0° C for 27 minutes. (to be freshly prepared and used).

(a) Direct method

Preparation of standard curve : Prepare 0.1% solution of pure cholesterol in chloroform. Pipette aliquots of 0.5, 0.6, 0.7, 0.8, 1.0, 1.1 and 1.2 ml in a graduated tube and makeup the volume to 3.0ml with chloroform. To each tube add 4.0ml of LB reagent and mix well. Incubate the contents at 25° C for 12 minutes in water bath. Quickly take optical density at 650 nm. Plot a graph between concentration and optical density.

Estimation : Take 5.0g sample and dissolve in 25ml chloroform. Pipette 1.0ml of this solution in a 15ml test tube. Add 2.0ml chloroform and 4.0ml LB reagent. Incubate at 25° C for 12 minutes and measure O.D. at 650 nm. Prepare a blank using 3.0ml chloroform and 4.0ml LB reagent. Calculate concentration from calibration curve. Report concentration of cholesterol as mg per 100g sample

Calculation

2ml solution gives concentration = A mg cholesterol

25ml solution gives concentration = A x 25 / 2 = B mg cholesterol (this represent mg cholesterol in 5g sample)

Total cholesterol (mg/100g) = Bx100/5

(b) Indirect method

(i) ***Extraction of unsaponifiable matter*** : Weigh 5g of ghee sample in a saponification flask. Add 40ml ethyl alcohol and 7ml of 50% KOH solution. Reflux contents for 30-40 minutes and then cool. Add 150 ml distilled water and transfer contents into separating funnel. Extract three times with 50ml portions of ethyl ether and collect extracts in another separating funnel. Wash ether extract with 2% aqueous KOH solution and then with water till alkali free. Filter ether layer through anhydrous sodium sulphate using Whatman No 40 filter paper. Evaporate the ether extract to dryness over water bath. Dissolve residue in 25ml glacial acetic acid. (solution A)

(ii) ***Preparation of standard curve*** : Prepare 0.1% solution of pure cholesterol in glacial acetic acid. Pipette aliquots of 0.1, 0.2, 0.3, 0.4, and 0.5 ml in a graduated tube and makeup the volume to 2.0ml with glacial acetic acid. To each tube add 4.0ml of LB reagent and mix well. Incubate the contents at 25° C for 35 minutes in water bath. Quickly take optical density at 650 nm. Plot a graph between concentration and optical density.

Estimation : Pipette 1.0 ml of solution A above in a glass stopped test tube.

Add 4.0 ml of freshly prepared LB reagent. Incubate at 25° C for 35 minutes and measure O.D. at 650 nm. Calculate concentration from calibration curve. Report concentration of cholesterol as mg per 100 g sample

Calculation

2ml solution gives concentration = A mg cholesterol

25ml solution gives concentration = A x 25 / 2 = B mg cholesterol (this represent mg cholesterol in 5 g sample)

Total cholesterol (mg/100 g) = Bx100/5

Antioxidant in Ghee (Qualitative test)

Reagent : Ehrlich reagent – Mix equal volume of 0.5% sodium nitrite solution and 0.5% sulfanilic acid solution containing conc. HCl; 72% ethyl alcohol ; 0.1N NaOH.

Procedure : Take 1 ml of melted fat in a test tube. Add 2 ml of 72% ethyl alcohol and shake well. Add 1 ml of Ehrlich reagent followed by 1 ml of 0.1N sodium hydroxide solution. Observe the colour of the mixture in tube.

Result

a) Development of red-purple colour indicates presence of BHA that shows maximum absorbance at 535 nm.

b) Development of distinct salmon pink colour indicates presence of BHT that shows maximum absorbance at 505 nm.

c) Development of yellow colour, which fades rapidly, indicates presence of propyl gallate that shows no measurable maximum in visible range.

Tests for Adultrants in Ghee

Higher cost of milk fat has caught the attention of unscrupulous elements for easy adulteration with cheaper quality vegetable oils and animal fats. Many tests have been developed for checking adulteration in ghee which are based on differences in nature and contents of major and minor components of milk fat and adulterants oils/fats. To confirm purity of milk fat, generally more than one test are employed as no single test can detect all types of adulterants.

1. Detection of vanaspati in ghee

(a) ***Baudouin test*** : Take 5ml of melted fat in a test tube. Add 5ml of conc. HCl and 0.2 g of sucrose. Mix well for one minute and keep undisturbed for 5 minutes. Appearance of crimson colour indicates presence of vanaspati. Add 5ml of distilled water and keep for 5 minutes. Persistence of crimson colour confirms the test.

(b) ***Furfural test*** : Take 5ml of melted fat in a test tube. Add 5ml of conc. HCl and 0.4 ml of 2% furfural solution in alcohol. Shake well and allow to separate the mixture, by keeping undisturbed for 5 minutes. Observe colour of acid layer. Appearance of pink/red colour indicates presence of vanaspati. Add 5 ml of distilled water, shake well and keep for 5 minutes. Persistence of red colour in acid layer confirms the test.

2. ***Detection of mineral oil*** : Take 1g of clarified fat in standard joint test tube. Add 5 ml of 0.5N ethanolic potassium hydroxide solution. Reflex the contents on boiling water bath for 10 minutes. Add 5 ml distilled water to saponified solution. Appearance of turbidity indicates presence of mineral oil.

3. ***Detection of animal body fat*** : Take 5g of melted sample in a test tube. Place in a water bath at 50 °C for 5 minutes. Replace tube in another water bath maintained at 23 °C. Record opacity time at regular interval using spectrophotometer. Note the time taken to acquire OD of 0.14-0.16 at 570 nm.

   Note : The opacity time for pure milk fat ranges from 12-18 minutes. Lesser time indicates presence of animal body fats. Higher time indicates presence of vegetable oils.

4. ***Detection of vegetable oils*** : Take 1-2 g of molten sample and dissolve in 2-3 ml of hexane. Add 1.5-2.0 ml of colour developing reagent (water, sulphuric acid, nitric acid in the ratio of 20:6:14).Shake vigorously and stand undisturbed until it separate into two layers. Appearance of distinct orange colour in upper layer indicates presence of vegetable oils.

   Note : Addition of 1ml each of 25% HCl & 5% sodium nitrile solution to hexane dissolved sample, shaking well and adding 1ml of 10% sodium hydroxide solution will give orange-red colour, indicating presence of Rice Bran Oil.

Suggested Readings

Acharya, K.T. (1997). Ghee, vanaspati and special fats in India. In: Lipid Technologies and applications. Ed. F.D.Gunstone and F.B.Padley, Marcel Dekker Inc., New York. pp 369-390.

Hamilton, R.J. and Rossell, J.B. (1986). Analysis of oils and fats. Elsevier Applied Science Publishers Ltd., London.

Indian Standards, IS:3508 (1966). Methods of sampling and tests for ghee. Manak Bhavan, Bahadur Shah Zafar Marg, New Delhi.

Lakshminarayanan, M. and Rama Murthi, M.K. (1985). Fractionation of buffalo milk fat and studies on physico-chemical properties. J.Dairy Science, 38(4): 256-264.

Lakshminarayanan, M. (1983). Fractionation of buffalo milk fat and studies on physico-chemical properties. Ph.D. Thesis, Kurukshetra University, Kurukshetra, Haryana.

Lakshminarayanan, M. and Rama Murthi, M.K.(1986). Cow and buffalo milk fat fraction: physico-chemical properties and fatty acid composition. J. Dairy Science, 39(3): 251-255.

Lal, D., Seth, R., Arora, K.L. and Ram, J. (1998). Detection of vegetable oil in milk fat. Indian Dairyman, 50(7):17-18.

Panda, D and Bindal, M.P. (1998). Detection of adulteration in ghee with animal fats and vegetable oils using opacity test. Indian J. Dairy Science, 50(2): 129-135.

Pandya, T.N. (1996). *Ghirt*. Ayurved Research J., 17(9):1-4.

Parodi, P.W. (1999). Milk fat components – possible chemopreventive agents for cancer and other diseases. Australian J. Dairy Technol., 51:24-32.

Saxena, R.B. and Daswani, M.T. (1996). Sturdy of Dairy *Ghirt*. Ayurved Research J., 17(9):8-10.

Sharma, R. and Singhal, O.P. (1995). Physico-chemical constants of ghee prepared from milk adulterated with forgein fats. Indian J. Dairy Sci. & Bio. Sci., 6:51-53.

Singh, K.P. and Singh, S.N. (1960). Variations in physico-chemical properties of ghee. Indian J. Dairy Science, 13: 143.

Singhal, O.P.(1980). Adulterants and methods of detection. Indian Dairyman, 32: 771-774.

Serunjogi, M.L., Abramsen, R.K. and Narvhus, J. (1998). Current knowledge of ghee and related products – a review. International Dairy J., 8(8):677-688.

Winton, A.L. and Winton, K.B. (1999). Techniques of food analysis. Allied Scientific Publishers, Bikaner, Rajasthan

Zaveri, K. (2000). Hridayrog. Bhansali trust, Surat, India.